Dr. Carol combines her expe[...] [barcode: M000016867] strong Christian faith to provide wise counsel for total wholeness for women in body, soul, and spirit. A book my wife wishes she had years ago! This is a valuable guide for husbands as well in understanding their wives' spiritual, emotional, and physical needs, feelings, and whole-person health care.

—PAUL KING, DMIN, DTH
FORMER PROFESSOR, ORAL ROBERTS UNIVERSITY
INTERDENOMINATIONAL INTERNATIONAL SPEAKER
AND SEMINAR TEACHER

Dr. Carol's guide fulfills an unmet need in the area of women's health. In a reader-friendly style the author combines medical science with her practical and personal experience through a Jesus Christ faith-based perspective. Dr. Carol's medical and ministry background gives her an extensive foundation from which to approach this subject. I enthusiastically endorse this book since it uniquely deals in a Christ-centered approach with difficult physical and mental/emotional health issues women face throughout the various stages of their lives. It will be a tremendous resource in women's health literature. I encourage the reader to go on this journey with *Dr. Carol's Guide to Women's Health*.

—DONALD R. TREDWAY, MD, PHD
FORMER CHAIRMAN OF THE DEPARTMENT OF OBSTETRICS AND
GYNECOLOGY AND UNIVERSITY OF
OKLAHOMA TULSA MEDICAL COLLEGE
RETIRED VICE PRESIDENT OF CLINICAL DEVELOPMENT UNIT,
METABOLIC AND REPRODUCTIVE ENDOCRINOLOGY,
EMD SERONO (MERCK KGA)

Dr. Carol Peters-Tanksley is not only a scholar and physician, but also a discerner of wisdom. *Dr. Carol's Guide to Women's Health* is a much-needed, valuable resource on women's health that offers not only practical information but also encouragement. This guide should be included in every church library, counselor's library, women's ministry library, and should be available as a reference tool for all women. The crucial information in this book has the potential to influence a healthier, holier, and more hopeful generation of women. I strongly recommend it.

—SHELLY BEACH

AWARD-WINNING AUTHOR, *THE SILENT SEDUCTION OF SELF-TALK*

MANAGING EDITOR, NIV HOPE IN THE MOURNING BIBLE

With degrees in both medicine (MD) and ministry (DMin), combined with years of experience, Dr. Carol has both the academic credentials and professional expertise to authoritatively address issues of women's health from a faith perspective. Her holistic approach and compassionate heart enable her to speak to a variety of concerns in a sensitive manner. Readers will feel as though they are having a private consultation with Dr. Carol as they interact with the wealth of material contained in this book.

—BILL BUKER, DMin, PhD, LPC

PROFESSOR OF COUNSELING, ORAL ROBERTS UNIVERSITY

Dr. Carol's Guide to Women's Health is a refreshingly positive guide for women throughout life's stages. Its holistic approach encourages women to take charge of their health and to make wise health-care choices. Her conversational style is patient-centered and fosters partnership with the women's health-care professional.

—JAMES S. POWERS, MD

ASSOCIATE PROFESSOR OF MEDICINE (GERIATRICS)

VANDERBILT UNIVERSITY SCHOOL OF MEDICINE

As the oldest health-cost-sharing ministry, we know that women often have their fear of health issues magnified because they see the topic as a mystery. When the mystery is reduced or removed, the road to health becomes a road of confidence and success. Healthy living is not just worthwhile but also possible. Step into the confidence needed to have a successful journey with this comprehensive, readable, and understandable guide to women's health written by a sojourner who knows the topic from inside and outside.

—REV. HOWARD S. RUSSELL

PRESIDENT AND CEO, CHRISTIAN HEALTHCARE MINISTRIES

Dr. Carol's insights into women's health will be a valuable resource for the women I help in their quest for healthy sexuality and spirituality. No question is too touchy for Dr. Carol. Her rich experience as a physician caring for women comes through to readers in a manner that both supports their faith and provides common sense. Each woman reading this will feel empowered to take charge of her health in every way. I gladly recommend this book for every woman who wants to live and feel better.

—SHANNON ETHRIDGE
LIFE/RELATIONSHIP COACH, SPEAKER, AND AUTHOR,
BEST-SELLING EVERY WOMAN'S BATTLE SERIES

Dr. Carol Peters-Tanksley has provided women of every age an incredible health resource. *Dr. Carol's Guide to Women's Health* is both easy to read and informative. Dr. Carol's holistic perspective on health gives women and girls the information they need to take control of their bodies and live healthier lives. I would recommend this book to any woman interested in bettering her own health or any mother interested in teaching her daughter about her developing body.

—MATTHEW S. STANFORD, PhD
CEO, HOPE AND HEALING CENTER AND INSTITUTE
AUTHOR, *GRACE FOR THE AFFLICTED: A CLINICAL AND BIBLICAL
PERSPECTIVE ON MENTAL ILLNESS*

Dr. Carol is in the unique position of having a deep understanding of women's health issues from an integrative medical and spiritual standpoint. *Dr. Carol's Guide to Women's Health* provides the reader with information, perspective, and guidance for issues where ethical or spiritual decisions impact women's health. Furthermore, her work speaks to the reader at a one-on-one level as though the reader were in a private consultation with Dr. Carol.

—SHAHRYAR K. KAVOUSSI, MD, MPH
REPRODUCTIVE ENDOCRINOLOGIST
AUSTIN FERTILITY AND REPRODUCTIVE MEDICINE

Bringing to her writing her experience as both a doctor of medicine and a doctor of ministry, Dr. Carol, in her book *Dr. Carol's Guide to Women's Health*, provides a reader-focused and comprehensive guide to healthy living in multiple areas of life for the woman of faith. Having shared the doctor of ministry experience with Dr. Carol, I can attest to her passion to help people experience the full and joyous life God calls us to physically, mentally, relationally, and spiritually.

—STEPHEN M STELLS, DMIN
FOUNDING PASTOR, HOUSE OF PRAYER
CHESTERFIELD, VIRGINIA

Completely Whole

Dr. Carol

Dr. Carol's Guide to

WOMEN'S
HEALTH

CAROL PETERS-TANKSLEY, MD, DMin

SILOAM

Most Charisma House Book Group products are available at special quantity discounts for bulk purchase for sales promotions, premiums, fund-raising, and educational needs. For details, write Charisma House Book Group, 600 Rinehart Road, Lake Mary, Florida 32746, or telephone (407) 333-0600.

Dr. Carol's Guide to Women's Health
   by Carol Peters-Tanksley, MD, DMin
Published by Siloam
Charisma Media/Charisma House Book Group
600 Rinehart Road
Lake Mary, Florida 32746
www.charismahouse.com

Cover design by Lisa Rae McClure
Design Director: Justin Evans

Visit the author's website at www.drcarolministries.com.

Library of Congress Cataloging-in-Publication Data:
An application to register this book for cataloging has been submitted to the Library of Congress.

International Standard Book Number: 978-1-62998-680-7
E-book ISBN: 978-1-62136-681-4

First edition

16 17 18 19 20 — 987654321
Printed in the United States of America

CONTENTS

Section 4: Mental and Emotional Health

ACKNOWLEDGMENTS

WHILE I HAVEN'T birthed any physical babies, bringing this book baby into the world makes me feel as though I can now say I've experienced pregnancy, labor, and delivery! And it would never have come into being without the invaluable support, contributions, and help of many others.

Thank you to Ann Byle, my literary agent, who has been like a godmother to this book baby and celebrated it as her own. And thank you to Tim Beals and Credo Communications for your invaluable influence in moving me from aspiring writer to published author.

Thank you to Jevon Bolden, former senior acquisitions editor at Charisma House, for seeing the future that this book baby could have. Your encouragement and experienced guidance has made this book baby so much better than it ever would have been. And thank you to the others at Charisma House who have been indispensable in bringing this book baby to life, especially Ann Mulchan and Debbie Marrie.

Thank you to my husband, Al Tanksley, who put up with many hours of loneliness and gave up many home-cooked meals while this book baby was being created. Your believing in me and this project has given me the courage and motivation to push through. You are, and always will be, the wind beneath my wings.

Most of all, thank You to Jesus, my Friend and Savior, for taking my own brokenness and turning it into something nourishing that can feed and bless others. May Your love and grace use these pages to bring hope, healing, and transformation to the women who read them.

And finally, thank you to the many women who trusted me to be their physician, friend, confidant, or counselor in some of the most intimate and challenging moments of their lives. Your stories, your resilience, and your refusal to settle for too little provide much of the fuel this book baby is built on. Carry on!

INTRODUCTION

I FACED THE LAST appointment of my day with very mixed emotions. Over many years of practice, I had experienced my share of difficult conversations with patients. But this time there was something bigger at stake.

Carrie and Justin were more than patients; they had become my friends. And my physician training and experience was no match for what they were coming in to discuss today. Even my years of theological training and ministry experience didn't provide much reassurance. This situation would require greater wisdom than I had, and I really didn't know what I was going to say.

Carrie had come to me some time ago for help with infertility, and along the way Justin had been closely involved as well. The months of treatment had proved difficult and frustrating. But a few weeks ago, everything seemed to be worth it. The pregnancy test read positive! It was a day for celebration mixed with hugs, tears, relief, anxiety, blood tests, and gratitude.

The joy didn't last long, however. Today Carrie and Justin were coming in to discuss some incredibly painful news. Recent tests indicated their much-prayed-for baby was affected by serious birth defects. Major organs were malformed. It was almost certain the child would not survive and develop long enough to be born, and if it did, there was no chance of life after birth. Carrie's obstetrician (another physician) was recommending immediate pregnancy termination.

Carrie and Justin struggled with that idea. They were both very educated and understood the implications of the ultrasound results. They also believed life is a gift from God. How could they voluntarily end the life of the child they had prayed so hard for? They had spent considerable time talking about their situation with the minister at their church. And still they struggled.

That's how I came to be sitting on my little rolling stool, looking across at two beautiful people facing one of the worst moments of their life together. They had talked with the doctors about all their questions. They had prayed with their minister. They had cried with their closest family members. But they needed help to bring all those pieces together in a way that would help them make the tough decisions in front of them.

Together we reviewed the medical facts and the test results. We talked about the risks, both known and unknown, to Carrie should she choose to continue the pregnancy. We addressed the emotional stress both Carrie and Justin were facing. We talked openly about the ethical and spiritual implications of whatever choice they might make and about issues such as fear, guilt, and grace. We tried to think through all of the choices they had, what they had control over, and what they didn't. We shed some tears. And we prayed together.

I didn't have any answers for Carrie and Justin that day. There was no magical medical intervention that would make Carrie's pregnancy normal. There was no 1-2-3 formula that would make their decision for them. There was no single Bible verse that would tell them all they needed to know.

Carrie and Justin didn't come that day for simple answers, although they would have gratefully accepted a simple answer if there had been one. They came for help in putting the medical, emotional, and spiritual aspects of this crisis together in a way that they could understand. (And yes, *understand* is far too tame and cerebral a word to describe what they needed.)

When they left the office that day, Carrie and Justin still faced some big decisions. Their pain was not over. They still had some unanswered questions. And their physical, emotional, and spiritual wounds were still raw. We agreed to stay in touch and to talk again if needed.

Carrie and Justin's story makes it clear how women's health is often a very complicated area. Yes, there are hormones, periods, pregnancy (or not), and menopause. But that's only one part of women's health. These physical dimensions of reproductive health often have great effects on a woman's mental and emotional health, her most intimate relationships, and even her spiritual health. And through it all a woman often struggles to deal with a sometimes confusing health-care system.

Their story also illustrates how women's health problems often include challenging ethical and moral issues. For a woman of faith these questions may be the most troublesome of all. While there are many sources of information on the medical aspects of such topics as contraception, infertility, and menopause, those sources don't usually include a faith perspective. It may seem difficult to bring together what you hear from your doctor and what you hear from your pastor, and to make appropriate decisions that take into account both medical science and your faith.

This book brings together medical science, my practical experience as a practicing physician, and a faith perspective. You won't find any theological pronouncements here, but I do use my theological and ministry experience to offer helpful insights I believe will be useful as you wrestle with your own health and health-care decisions.

This book is designed to be a guide that will help you put the medical, emotional, and spiritual components of your health in some kind of perspective. Think of me sitting across from you on my little rolling stool, explaining the different aspects of your health, answering your questions, helping you understand what you can do to help yourself, and considering God's perspective on the decisions you may need to make.

Some chapters will focus almost entirely on your physical health, what you can do on your own to be healthier, and what medical treatments you might consider. These chapters will only address ethical or spiritual issues where necessary. Some chapters will focus on interacting with today's complex health-care system. Others will more directly address emotional and spiritual health.

You may not find every chapter equally helpful for your own situation. Feel free to skim over the areas that don't apply to you and spend more time on the areas where you need more understanding. This book is not intended to provide medical care or to diagnose or treat any medical illness or condition. Please use the information here to see what steps you can take to maximize your own health, and then talk with your own physician.

What about Carrie and Justin? I don't know what decision they made or would have made. Carrie called me not long after our meeting to tell me, "God answered our prayer. I'm having a miscarriage."

That may not seem like an answer to you, but it was to Carrie and Justin. They believe God honored their faith such that they were not forced to make a decision they didn't want to have to make. And they were terribly grateful.

No single book can answer all your questions about health. You may be faced with some decisions this book doesn't directly address. You may not experience answers in the same way Carrie and Justin did. But the ideas and principles discussed here will provide you with insight and guidance, whatever challenging health issues you may face.

I pray these pages help you experience a life full of understanding, confidence, and joy as you live healthfully in body, mind, and soul.

Chapter 1
WHAT IS A HEALTHY WOMAN?

ARE YOU HEALTHY? How healthy are you? If you were to walk through some magical doorway that made you instantly and completely healthy, would you recognize yourself? What would be different about you then compared to the person you are right now?

Thankfully we've come a long way from the idea that health is simply the absence of disease. Health involves our ability to function at our best in every area of our lives. It doesn't happen by accident. As with most good things, the more intentional you are about understanding and taking responsibility for your health, the better the outcome you will achieve.

Women's health has become a hot topic in twenty-first-century culture. When you hear that term—*women's health*—you probably think first of the kind of health care you would receive at a women's clinic or your ob-gyn physician's office. And there are plenty of people who have made women's health a topic of political and social controversy. In some ways that's been a good thing. The controversies have brought some of the issues into the light.

But in other ways the controversies over such things as contraception, abortion, and insurance coverage have obscured what women's health is really all about. A healthy woman is so much more than her reproductive organs. We do all women a disservice when we forget that.

Let's begin by looking at what a healthy woman—and therefore women's health—is all about.

AN INTEGRATIVE VIEW OF HEALTH

Imagine the ideal woman in your mind. Oh, I know the popular media has idealized the skinny, teenage body with long hair, long legs, and large breasts. But let's get real for a moment. Try your best to get that Barbie picture out of your mind and imagine what a healthy woman would look like. Picture a woman the age you are right now, since you can't undo your birthdays.

Certainly your ideal woman wouldn't be sick, but that would only be

1

a start. I'm sure you picture her looking healthy in every way. She would have bright, clear eyes that sparkle when she looks at you. Her skin would be glowing, and her hair would look alive. She would be at a healthy weight. Her body would be strong, fully rested, and full of energy.

A woman can't look that way physically on the outside without being healthy on the inside. Rest, nutrition, and exercise certainly help. But her mental state makes a difference as well. You'd be able to tell right away if she were anxious, depressed, stressed, or worried, or even if she were feeling worked over by her hormones. You could get a good idea of what she was thinking about just from the look on her face.

Relationships also affect the way your ideal woman looks and feels. If you aren't sure about that, just look at the women in line the next time you go to the grocery store or sit in a doctor's office. Imagine what kind of personal relationships each woman has. You might see the anxious and angry divorcée, the happy grandmother married to the same man for fifty years, or the single businesswoman secretly hungry for a boyfriend. You might be wrong in what you imagine for each person, but the exercise shows you how much your relationships show in your face and behavior.

You can also tell a lot about your ideal woman's spiritual life by looking at her. Is she weighed down by guilt or shame? Is she anxious about what God thinks of her? Is she careless about the impact of her behavior on others? Does she feel her life has a purpose? Is she living with peace, joy, and love?

I hope you can see from this discussion how much each aspect of a woman's life impacts every other area. If you're sick physically, your emotions will be more difficult to handle. If your marriage is a mess, your body will be stressed. Whatever you do to get healthier in one area will positively benefit your health in every other area as well.

Understanding this integrative view of women's health is so important. Women of faith sometimes struggle here. On one hand, focusing on the eternal importance of one's spiritual life has led some to ignore the importance of developing a healthy lifestyle, healthy thinking, and healthy relationships. Likewise, some have made their physical health a primary goal without addressing the other dimensions of health that both affect and are affected by our physical well-being.

As a Christian woman, you have even more reason to take your health seriously. God made you spirit, soul, and body. He redeemed you spirit, soul, and body. His Holy Spirit makes your body His temple

(1 Cor. 6:19–20). And His plan for you is that "your whole spirit, soul and body be kept blameless at the coming of our Lord Jesus Christ" (1 Thess. 5:23). God cares about your health, and you honor Him by caring about it as well.

Best of all, the ideal woman you imagined can be you. While you can't entirely escape sickness or aging in this life, you can certainly slow them down. Too many women settle for too little. They accept being sick, tired, and miserable as normal. They may look to a pill, a specific diet, a new relationship, or an expensive program to make them feel better. Sometimes some of those things are necessary. But much more often what's needed is simply for you to take charge of your health.

TAKE CHARGE

Recently I was asked to perform a consultation on a sixty-one-year-old lady I'll call Sarah who was hospitalized with multiple problems. She had chronic obstructive pulmonary disease, sleep apnea, diabetes, and kidney failure. She had just returned from the cardiac suite after having an angioplasty for a small heart attack. She couldn't walk without assistance, and her list of medications would keep a pharmacy in business. Her daughter had noticed some minimal vaginal spotting, which was the reason for my consultation.

As I read Sarah's chart, her primary physician's comment seemed so sad: "The patient and her family demonstrate no real interest in taking action to improve her health." And after meeting with Sarah and her daughter, I could make a definite prediction: in twenty-five years, this patient's daughter would be in the same physical state as her mother unless she made some dramatic changes.

None of that is necessary. There isn't one of this patient's problems that could not have been prevented by making some fairly modest lifestyle changes. And each one of her problems could be significantly improved by making some relatively simple changes right now. But she and her family aren't interested. Instead, she will probably die soon. How tragic!

I don't want you to end up like Sarah. In one twenty-minute consultation, I could do very little to stimulate Sarah to take charge of her health. But you're reading this book. You're taking your health seriously. You know there are things you need to know, understand, and do if you want to look, feel, and function at your best. And if you do that, I can promise you that I won't be writing this about you when you're sixty-one!

If you're interested in feeling better, living longer, and being healthier in every way, here are some of the things you can do to take charge of your health and your health care:

+ Accept the reality that your health is your responsibility, not that of your parents, your doctor, the government, or anyone else.

+ Be intellectually hungry for information about things that impact your health.

+ Be willing to examine your life for habits or behaviors that might be negatively impacting your health.

+ Use the tools and information you find to actually make changes that will improve your health.

+ Thoughtfully ask questions of health-care professionals about things you don't know or understand.

+ Become an informed consumer of health care, including medical tests, medications, supplements, and insurance alternatives.

+ Think about your thinking, and practice healthier thinking in areas where you struggle.

+ Search out professionals when you need extra help, and see yourself as a partner with them in making decisions and taking action.

+ See yourself and God as working together for your maximum well-being in every area of your life.

Nobody else will ever care more about you and your health than you do. And if they do, it won't do you any good. It's your body, your health, your health care, your pocketbook, and your life that we're talking about. You get to choose what to do about it. Own it all, and I guarantee you'll be healthier than if you let anyone else take that responsibility from you.

WHAT WOULD HEALTHY LOOK LIKE?

While driving through a major US city, I scanned the channels on the radio. The host of a locally popular talk show was promoting healthy living by focusing on natural foods and supplements. She was a breast cancer survivor, and her passion to help others gain physical health was obvious.

Then she made a comment that shocked me. "I take over sixty pills a day, all of them supplements," she said. "I take no medications."

Now the idea of *natural* is a good one. I love natural! But sixty pills a day? There is absolutely no way even the most brilliant scientist, doctor, or nutritionist can tell you what effect that amount and variety of substances will have on your body. This is not about science. This is not about natural. This is about a desperation to be healthy.

I can sympathize with this talk-show host. Surviving cancer gives you a whole different perspective on life. When you've been sick, many people will do just about anything to regain their physical health. But sixty pills a day is not the answer. (OK, if you've had a heart transplant or have some other terribly serious condition, perhaps that many pills might be necessary.)

If you aim at nothing, you'll reach it every time. You can't be nineteen forever. (And would you really want to be?) And you don't want to end up like Sarah. So it's worth considering what being healthy would really look like.

Here's a realistic picture of health that's worth aiming for:

- **Fully alive physically.** You feel generally strong and energetic a majority of the time. You have no preventable lifestyle illnesses and are free from destructive lifestyle behaviors, such as substance abuse and unhealthy sexual behavior. You give your body an appropriate degree of tender loving care without making it the definition of who you are. You have the physical ability to fully engage in the work or vocation that fulfills the purpose God has for you.

- **Fully alive mentally and emotionally.** You're able to experience the full range of human emotions—sadness, grief, pain, joy, love, hope, and more. You aren't stuck in a constant state of anger, fear, anxiety, bitterness, or other destructive emotions. You're able to choose what to think about and take personal responsibility for your thoughts and emotions.

- **Fully alive relationally.** If you're married, your relationship with your spouse is characterized by mutual love and respect. If you're single, you're living a full and vibrant life connected with others in healthy ways. You have a full range of relationships with other people characterized by mutuality, love, and growth. You seek out ways to benefit the lives of others while keeping your own heart full.

+ **Fully alive spiritually.** You have a relationship with God that is resilient, growing, and real. You continue to experience God's transforming power in all aspects of your life. You demonstrate hope for the future in the middle of troubles now. You care about your heart and protect it with everything you have (Prov. 4:23). Your spiritual life provides a positive benefit to your physical, emotional, and relational health as well.

Being healthy is not synonymous with youth or beauty. It's not something you spend exorbitant amounts of money to attain, and it doesn't go away the moment you feel tired or need a prescription. It's not available only to those who have the perfect genetics or spend hours in the gym.

Being healthy means being fully alive in every area of your being, taking charge of what's in your control, and using all the resources you have available to handle challenges that inevitably come along. It's being the best *you* that you can be.

How You See Yourself

Self-image has become an overused buzzword, but it expresses a vitally important concept. As Henry Ford is credited with saying, "Whether you think you can or think you can't, you're right." Take a moment right now and write down at least twenty words that you would use to describe yourself. Go ahead. Push yourself. I would guess that you can come up with a few quite easily but that it will become more difficult as you go along.

Here are some words you might use: *Pretty. Plain. Overworked. Resilient. Strong. Lonely. Fat. Confused. Unheard. Brash. Happy. Communicative. Smart. Connected. Youthful. Skinny. Tired. Shameful. Anxious. Lovely. Desirable. Distracted. Hopeful. Powerless. Weary. Fit. Old. Studious. Energetic. Creative. Healthy. Driven. Persistent. Caring. Loved. Mature. Frustrated. Graceful. Feminine. Powerful. Wise.*

Have you created your list? How well does it describe how you see yourself? How well do you think it describes the real you?

God sees you as you are now, but He also sees you as He created you to be and as you can become. This exercise is designed to help you do the same and to show you how powerful your self-image is in relation to your health. If you really want to make this exercise powerful, create a second list of twenty words describing yourself five years from now. Are they different?

If you see yourself as tired, powerless, and old, you may easily become bitter at how life has done you wrong. You'll look for others to fix you and become frustrated and angry when they won't or can't do so. You won't take charge of your health. And I can promise you that in five years, you'll look and feel older, sicker, and more miserable than you do right now.

If, however, you see yourself as resilient, creative, and wise, you will almost certainly look and feel stronger and healthier in five years than you do right now. You'll take charge of your health and gratefully use resources to help you live and feel better. Your future will certainly present challenges, but you'll be up to the task. Your joy can increase regardless of what life brings.

I encourage you to choose the way in which you see yourself. None of us can do this perfectly, but you can become better at it. Surround yourself with positive people, high-quality resources, and well-chosen professionals when you need them. For women of faith, God's Word provides perhaps the best source of encouragement, wisdom, and truth available in this area. All these steps will help you see yourself as taking charge of your health, and as a result you'll become increasingly better at doing so.

DON'T DO IT ALONE

Human beings are created for community, and we as women are perhaps especially needy in this area. The kinds of relationships you cultivate will make a huge difference in how helpful this book is to you and how healthy you are in the months and years ahead.

Here are a few ways you can become healthier through the people you spend time with:

+ You can go walking regularly with a girlfriend.
+ You can connect with other women who are facing a similar health problem as you are.

+ You can work out a helpful signal with your husband to help
  you stop negative talking or thinking right away.
+ You can talk about helpful ways to shop for and prepare
  healthful food with your coworkers or women's study group.
+ You can invest in a volunteer opportunity or church group that
  brings you meaning and joy.
+ You can open yourself to professional help when you need
  it, whether it be doctors, counselors, nutrition experts, or
  pastors.

There will always be people who know more than you do in certain areas. That's a good thing; take advantage of their knowledge and experience. That's part of what professionals are for, but it's also a benefit of connecting with others in many contexts. And when you can find other women to connect with who are also working toward being fully alive—healthy—in every area of their lives, you are blessed indeed.

Where does spirituality fit into becoming healthier? There's a whole chapter on healthy spirituality near the end of this book. If you're a woman of faith, remember that God cares about your health. His presence in your life will make a difference at every stage of your journey. Investing in a relationship with Him is the most important part of not doing it alone.

So let's jump right into the areas of women's health that you're most likely concerned about. Here I sit on my little rolling stool, ready to answer your questions and help guide you through the fascinating journey of becoming a healthy woman. Get ready to take charge of your health and your health care.

Section 1

REPRODUCTIVE HEALTH

Chapter 2

WHAT'S NORMAL AND WHAT'S NOT

WHEN AN OLD Aretha Franklin song comes on the air, some of us can feel like shouting about the need we have for R-E-S-P-E-C-T or how something or someone can make us feel like a natural woman. Being a woman can be glorious and fulfilling. That's the way we were meant to be. We're strong yet sometimes vulnerable, resilient yet sometimes broken.

There are times being a woman can also be painful and frustrating. The uniqueness we experience as women is especially evident during the nearly forty years of our lives we spend dealing with hormonal ups and downs, periods, pregnancy (or not), birth control (or not), and all the associated physical and emotional ways our femininity displays itself. I've helped women deal with these both fulfilling and challenging aspects of their womanly selves for well over twenty years, and I am looking forward to doing the same with you.

Many would agree that throughout the centuries, women have experienced more than their share of oppression. In our modern world women continue to earn less than men in most circumstances. Domestic violence and sexual violence bring heartache and trauma to too many. It's understandable that many women feel controlled, pushed down, and even victimized.

Many positive changes have happened in the lives of women over the past several decades, but the most important change that must happen is in how we see ourselves. You are only a victim if you choose to be one. That is true in every area of life, but as it relates to the topic of this book, it is especially true in the area of your health. Much of this book will help you find the understanding and tools to take charge of your health in every way.

What that looks like varies during different periods of a woman's life. Understanding what's normal for the life stage you're in now is the first step in taking charge of your health.

PUBERTY

Somewhere around age seven or eight, something begins to awaken in a young girl's brain. Nothing has changed on the outside yet, but the part of her central nervous system that will control her reproductive life for the next forty years begins to function. Specific brain cells in the hypothalamus "wake up" and start producing signals and hormones, which then make their way to the pituitary gland. We don't know specifically what it is that turns on this part of the central nervous system; it's one of the glorious mysteries of creation.

For most girls, the first physical sign of puberty is breast budding—a small, sometimes tender "lump" under the nipple. That's an indication the hypothalamus, pituitary gland, and ovaries are all beginning to function and that estrogen is being produced. The average age for a girl's first breast development is nine to ten years old, though that can vary a lot. Some girls notice pubic hair as the first physical sign of puberty. The average age at which girls enter puberty has decreased over the last several decades, possibly because of factors in our environment, the quality of our food, and the frequency of childhood obesity.

The slowly increasing estrogen levels during puberty accomplish a number of things. Estrogen stimulates a girl's bones to grow rapidly, causing a growth spurt. Breast tissue continues to enlarge. Pubic hair increases. And, finally, menstruation begins. The average age for menarche—a girl's first period—is twelve, although that also varies quite a bit. The development of physical changes from first noticing early breast development until a girl's first period usually takes a couple years.

Health Tip

The age of normal puberty varies a lot. It's time to see a doctor if:

- *Physical signs of puberty begin prior to age eight.*
- *There are no physical signs of puberty by age thirteen.*
- *Periods have not started by age fifteen.*

Anxiety around body image is just one of the challenges girls experience as they go through the transition from girlhood to womanhood. Going through puberty earlier or later than one's peers can be a big source of concern. Occasionally early or late puberty is a sign of a serious medical condition. If a girl shows physical signs of puberty before age eight, if she has not shown any signs of puberty at all by age thirteen, or if she has been showing external signs of puberty but has not had a period by age fifteen, it's time to see a doctor. Nothing may be wrong, but it's worth checking out.

During the first several years after menarche, irregular periods are quite common. Although a girl may ovulate with her very first period, it usually takes a few years for her whole reproductive system to fully mature. This is a good time to begin keeping track of menstrual cycles. This habit will be helpful in many ways for many years to come.

A menstrual calendar can be helpful for understanding what's normal for you, and it can also be very helpful whenever you see your doctor. A simple calendar, such as the one provided, works just fine. Place a checkmark or dot in the box when you have a day of light bleeding, and fill in the box when you have a heavy day. Many young women now use period tracker apps on their smartphones. There are dozens available. Here are several for which I've received good feedback or recommendations:

- Glow: available for Apple devices (www.glowing.com)
- Period Tracker Lite: available for Android and Apple devices
- Pink Pad: available for Android and Apple devices (www .pinkp.ad)
- Fertility Friend: available for Apple devices (www.fertility friend.com)
- CycleBeads: available for Android and Apple devices (www .cyclebeads.com)

These apps are all free or have a free version. Some have extra features available in a paid version.

Some young women find their periods to be especially heavy or painful during the first few years after menarche. There are a few things you can do on your own to make your periods less problematic. Being overweight makes these problems worse for some young women, so eating healthy and getting regular exercise is especially important. (See chapters 9 and 10 for more on this.) That may seem like a small thing, but it's not. Extra weight affects many things about your female hormones, and it's worth working hard to keep it under control.

Regular exercise such as running, swimming, cycling, or team sports may improve menstrual cramps significantly and is enough to stop them completely in some women. Also, constipation around the time of your period may make it all even worse. Exercise, drinking plenty of water, and eating more fruits and vegetables can lessen how troublesome this becomes. A heating pad or a warm bath or shower can also help keep menstrual cramps under control.

Menstrual Cycle Record

YEAR:

Month	1	2	3	4	5	6	7	8	9	10	11	12	13	14	15	16	17	18	19	20	21	22	23	24	25	26	27	28	29	30	31
Jan.																															■
Feb.																													■	■	■
Mar.																															
Apr.																															■
May																															
June																															■
July																															
Aug.																															
Sept.																															■
Oct.																															
Nov.																															■
Dec.																															

NORMAL PERIODS

From age twelve through age fifty the average woman will have more than four hundred periods. In a normal cycle a few of the eggs in a woman's ovaries become available during any given month. The hormone signals from the pituitary gland (primarily FSH, follicle stimulating hormone) encourage those eggs to continue to develop. Approximately a week prior to ovulation, one of those eggs becomes queen and continues to grow while the others deteriorate. Once that egg is mature, it is released from the ovary—the moment of ovulation. While the egg has been developing, the ovary has also been producing estrogen, which causes the lining of the uterus to become thick and lush.

After the egg is released, the cells left in the ovary develop into a structure called the corpus luteum and begin to produce progesterone. No ovulation, no progesterone. During the twelve days or so that progesterone is produced, the lining of the uterus becomes mature in preparation for an embryo to attach, should pregnancy occur. If pregnancy does not happen, the levels of estrogen and progesterone decrease, triggering the onset of menstrual bleeding. The time from ovulation to the following menstrual period is quite consistent at thirteen to fourteen days. The following month, another group of eggs becomes available, and the cycle begins again.

Health Tip

A "normal" period:

- *Begins about every four weeks*
- *Lasts four to seven days in total*
- *Brings moderate bleeding for a couple days and then lessens*
- *May be associated with mild pelvic cramping or pressure*

All those periods during a woman's reproductive life involve a lot of pads or tampons and a lot of "hormonal" days. Some women have barely a hiccup in their daily lives when their period comes each month. It begins predictably, exactly four weeks after the last one, and brings very little discomfort. The first day or two involves moderate bleeding, during which a new pad or tampon is needed about every three or four hours, followed by another three or four days of gradually decreasing bleeding. While there's a significant variation in "normal" from woman to woman, if this describes your periods, they're probably normal.

ABNORMAL PERIODS

A number of things can disrupt this monthly rise and fall of hormones. This whole ovulation process is controlled by the hypothalamus at the base of the brain. This vital brain area has connections with many other brain areas. Anything that affects the central nervous system can potentially disrupt ovulation. Stress can do so. For example, we know that college students often have delayed or absent periods during final exams or other stressful times. Many medical illnesses, including thyroid disease, kidney disease, diabetes, and others, may also disrupt menstrual periods at times. So can a number of medications.

For some women every menstrual period brings a major disruption in her life and well-being. Physical and mental discomfort begin days prior to her period. Serious cramping pain may begin even before bleeding comes. Bleeding is heavy, necessitating a new pad or tampon every hour or two for a few days. Symptoms may be so bad she spends a day or two home from work or school each month. Bleeding may last for more than a week, and the whole process may disrupt her life for ten days or more every month.

The range of "normal" is wide when it comes to women and their periods, but that doesn't mean you have to put up with misery. There are almost always things you can do to make your monthly cycle manageable, either on your own or with medical treatment. Too often I see women put up with disabling symptoms that are completely unnecessary.

Should your period be painful? A mild to moderate sensation of pelvic pressure or cramping pain for a day or two is probably normal. Raspberry tea may help menstrual cramps for some women. Regular exercise, such as swimming, running, or cycling, may also significantly help menstrual pain. Over-the-counter medications such as acetaminophen, ibuprofen, or naproxen may be very effective. They work best when started before pain becomes severe. The hormonal changes during your period trigger the production of prostaglandins, substances that cause muscle spasms and changes in blood flow to the pelvic organs. If you commonly have pain during your period, taking ibuprofen at the first sign of either cramps or bleeding will drastically slow down the production of those prostaglandins and may prevent pain in many cases.

If the pain with your period is enough to disrupt your life significantly or if these simple measures don't control your pain relatively easily, it's time to see a doctor. Mild pain with periods is OK. Severe pain is *not* OK and may signal a more significant medical problem, such as endometriosis or pelvic inflammatory disease.

What about diet and periods? Drinking plenty of fluids and eating a diet rich in fruits and vegetables (which are full of antioxidants and fiber) may lessen some of the symptoms around your period. Some women find that difficult bowel movements or constipation become worse around their periods, and extra fluid and fiber can improve these symptoms.

PMS

Most women with ovulatory menstrual cycles have at least one symptom of premenstrual syndrome, or PMS. Symptoms may be physical, such as bloating, water retention, acne, trouble sleeping, food cravings, backache, headache, muscle aches, or breast pain. Symptoms may also be mental, such as trouble concentrating, irritability, anxiety, mood swings, depression, crying spells, or being easily angered.

I've been asked many times to measure hormone blood levels in women with PMS to find out what's missing or out of balance. The truth is that no blood test can diagnose PMS. The symptoms aren't caused by an abnormal level of any hormone or by an abnormal balance between hormones. Some health practitioners have described *estrogen dominant* or *progesterone dominant* types of symptoms. Unfortunately those categories are not supported by good research and are not useful in helping women manage their symptoms.

What causes symptoms of PMS is the rise and fall of ovarian

Health Tip

To improve difficult or painful periods:

- *Drink plenty of water.*
- *Get regular exercise.*
- *Eat plenty of fiber (especially in fruits and vegetables).*
- *Try raspberry tea.*
- *Try acetaminophen, ibuprofen, or naproxen.*

hormones, especially estrogen and progesterone. Those hormones change significantly from day to day and even hour to hour during the time between ovulation and a woman's next period. When those hormones are not fluctuating (such as before puberty, during pregnancy, or after menopause), there's no PMS.

For many women PMS is nothing more than a gentle reminder that their menstrual period is on its way. The symptoms don't disrupt their daily life significantly, and they resolve quickly once menstrual bleeding begins. For others the symptoms become severe and even disabling. The good news is that there are many things that can help lessen these symptoms. We'll talk a lot more about PMS and what to do about it in chapter 20.

Normal Menopause

Somewhere around age fifty your ovaries just don't have any more eggs. Once those eggs are gone, estrogen production from the ovaries drops dramatically, by about 90 percent. Testosterone production also drops, though less dramatically—about 50 percent. (Yes, women's ovaries make some testosterone too.)

During the last several years of a woman's reproductive life, ovulation becomes less and less predictable. Menstrual periods become less regular. Some women experience periods that become progressively lighter and farther apart until they simply stop. Other women experience periods that become heavier, longer, and closer together before stopping. The average woman experiences three to five years of these menstrual changes before her final period, which occurs, on average, at age fifty-one.

The average age of a woman's last period varies considerably. If you know when your mother, aunts, or older sisters experienced menopause, you'll have a pretty good idea of when to expect it yourself. If a woman's ovaries stop functioning before age forty, she is considered to have premature menopause (premature ovarian failure), which may also be associated with other medical problems. At the other end of the spectrum, it's very rare for a woman to still be having periods in her late fifties. Many of the cycles a woman has during the last few years before menopause are often anovulatory, meaning no mature egg is released from the ovary. That is in part why her cycles become much less predictable.

Smoking leads to earlier menopause, as tobacco damages the eggs and surrounding follicles in the ovaries. Ovarian surgery, chemotherapy, and certain other serious illnesses may also lead to earlier menopause.

The swings in reproductive hormone levels are much more dramatic in the years approaching menopause than they were during a woman's twenties and thirties. The peak estrogen levels may be higher, and the lows may be lower. Progesterone production becomes less predictable. These more dramatic hormone swings each month may be why some women have worsening symptoms of PMS during these years. This may also be why some women begin having hot flashes and night sweats even while they are still having periods.

It's impossible to predict exactly when a woman's last period will be. Blood tests, including tests for FSH (follicle stimulating hormone) and MIH (mullerian inhibiting factor or hormone), may give some indication as to whether a woman is going through the menopause transition. But only after one year has passed with no menstrual periods is a woman said to be truly menopausal.

This is only a brief overview of what happens during the menopause transition. Chapter 8 is devoted entirely to this important topic, including ways to manage the symptoms and what may be abnormal.

By now, you probably have a pretty good idea about whether your experience is normal or abnormal when it comes to reproductive health. But what if it's not normal? In the next two chapters, we'll talk specifically about various conditions related to pelvic pain, abnormal menstrual bleeding, and more.

A Few Questions

At the end of each chapter I've included a few questions on the chapter's subject that I often receive. You may wonder about some of the matters posed here too.

Q: Is it OK to wear tampons?

A: Usually yes. In most cases, whether you wear a tampon or a pad is completely a personal choice. If you've recently delivered a baby or had pelvic surgery, your doctor will ask you to not put anything in the vagina, including a tampon, for a period of time. If you are being treated for a vaginal or pelvic infection, it is usually better to avoid tampons temporarily.

Toxic shock syndrome (TSS) is quite rare and usually only occurs with the use of superabsorbent tampons that are left in too long. The biggest thing to worry about is forgetting to take a tampon out at the end of your period. Think of a reminder that works for you, such as an alert on your smartphone or a checkmark on your calendar. Or don't put away your tampon box until you've taken out the last one for that month. Use something to remind you to be sure you haven't forgotten one inside.

Q: Is it OK to have sex during my menstrual period?

A: Some women (and their partners) may feel uncomfortable having sex during times of menstrual bleeding. But medically speaking, there's no need to avoid intercourse during your period if both of you want to do so.

Q: Can I exercise (including swimming) during my menstrual period?

A: Yes! Physical exercise even while on your period is a great way to lessen both the physical and emotional tension some women experience. To lessen the risk of "accidents," some women may choose to use tampons during certain forms of exercise (such as swimming) even if they use pads during the rest of their period. Staying active, even during your period, is one of the most important ways to stay healthy and feel better.

Q: I have a vaginal discharge. Is this normal?

A: The glands in the cervix and the vaginal tissues normally secrete a small amount of clear or white liquid. Healthy bacteria, principally lactobacilli, also thrive in the healthy vagina. You need some moisture to keep the vagina comfortable and healthy. If it were dry, you'd be miserable. (Just ask some postmenopausal women!) Sometimes this vaginal moisture is enough to notice as secretions on your underwear or a minipad.

Vaginal discharge is abnormal when it is gray, green, yellow, or bloody; when it is excessive in amount; or when it is associated with a foul or fishy odor. If you also have itching, irritation, or pain, a vaginal discharge may indicate some type of infection. See your doctor in these cases.

Q: Should I douche?

A: Generally, no. Douching after intercourse does not decrease the chance of pregnancy or a sexually transmitted infection. Douching after a menstrual period is not necessary; the normal vaginal secretions effectively remove any remaining menstrual blood quite quickly. Instead of improving vaginal health, douching removes much of the healthy lactobacilli and may increase the chance of a vaginal infection.

Q: I've heard about some women being estrogen dominant or progesterone dominant. Should I worry about this?

A: No. These terms have been made popular by promoters of certain health products or programs and have no valid scientific basis. The most common claim is that certain blood or saliva tests will determine which hormone you lack so you can be sold a certain product. Buyer beware!

If you aren't ovulating normally, your ovaries aren't making progesterone. However, simply taking progesterone won't solve your problem. You need to find out why you aren't ovulating. Fat tissue always makes extra estrogen, but that doesn't mean taking progesterone will solve your weight problem. Lose weight, and the extra estrogen will take care of itself.

Chapter 3

WHEN IT'S NOT NORMAL
PART 1: PAIN

I THINK IT'S TRUE that women are the stronger sex. (Just think how many babies would not be born if men were the ones who had to go through labor!) Many women go on living and functioning even while they are experiencing pain. Women are incredibly strong.

Dealing with any pain, however, is often very debilitating. I don't know about you, but I hate pain. And pelvic pain is one of the more debilitating problems too many women struggle with. It's certainly one of the most frequent problems for which women seek care from a gynecologist. Pelvic pain affects a woman's ability to enjoy life, to work, and to offer her best self to her family and others. It impacts her most intimate relationships and her total quality of life.

The good news is that pain is often unnecessary. That doesn't mean one magic treatment can always take away pain forever. But so many women suffer needlessly when their pain could have been helped. Don't be one of them!

To begin, it's important to pay attention to when you experience pain. As far as pelvic pain goes, there are three principal questions to ask:

+ Does the pain seem to be related to your periods?
+ Does the pain occur with intercourse?
+ Is the pain unrelated to either of the above?

Anything else you notice about the timing of your pain can also be helpful.

If you're struggling with pelvic pain, here are some conditions that may be affecting you.

ENDOMETRIOSIS

The uterine lining—the endometrium—is naturally designed to bleed every month when a woman has a period. In a woman with endometriosis, bits of that same kind of tissue grow in other places outside the uterine cavity. Most often these growths, or implants, as they are called, are present around the ovaries, the outside of the uterus, or other organs in the pelvic area, such as the bladder, colon, or tissue lining the pelvic cavity. More rarely, these growths appear in other areas of the body.

Endometriosis implants respond to hormones in a similar way as the endometrium: estrogen makes them grow, and progesterone makes them stop growing. When the uterine lining bleeds, these implants may bleed a little also. That blood has nowhere to go and sometimes may collect inside the ovary or lead to free blood inside the pelvis. That blood can cause significant pain and can lead to scar tissue in the areas where the implants are located. This is a somewhat simplified description of endometriosis, but it's a picture you can get your mind around. Remembering this description will help you understand a lot about what helps endometriosis and how treatments work.

Endometriosis affects millions of women, and it can occur at any age, from a girl's first period through menopause. The most common symptom of endometriosis is pain, sometimes severe. The pain is usually concentrated around the time of your menstrual period and may be absent the rest of the month. Women with endometriosis usually know their period is on its way because significant pelvic pain begins first, sometimes a day or two prior to bleeding. Pain with intercourse is also common, and pain may be present throughout the entire month.

Your periods may be heavier or irregular if you have endometriosis. Spotting and pelvic pain may begin a day or two prior to menstrual bleeding. Endometriosis may also cause infertility, as endometriosis implants are thought to make the pelvic environment unhealthy for embryos. Severe endometriosis may also cause scar tissue that damages the ovaries and fallopian tubes. More severe endometriosis may also cause pain or bleeding with bowel movements, pain or bleeding with urination, bloating, nausea, or other symptoms.

Endometriosis is not a lifestyle illness. There's essentially nothing you can do to cause it or to prevent it. There is, however, a genetic component to endometriosis. If other female family members, such as your mother, sister, or aunt, have had the disorder, it increases the likelihood you may have it also.

If you have severe pain with your periods or experience pelvic pain with any of the other above-mentioned symptoms, it's time to be evaluated for endometriosis. Many women may have this disorder without knowing it because they haven't had an appropriate medical evaluation.

A pelvic exam and an ultrasound may give your doctor clues about the likelihood that your pain is caused by endometriosis, but those measures can't make the diagnosis. Sometimes blood tests, including CA125, are also used, but they can't make the diagnosis either.

The only way you and your doctor can know for sure whether or not you have endometriosis is through a laparoscopy, so-called *belly-button surgery*, to look inside the abdomen and pelvis. The implants of endometriosis look quite characteristic at the time of laparoscopy, and

<table><tr><td>**Health Tip**</td></tr><tr><td>*The only way to diagnose endometriosis is via laparoscopy. However, it's often helpful to treat pain as though it were endometriosis, even without a certain diagnosis.*</td></tr></table>

your doctor may also take biopsies of suspicious areas if there's any question. The other helpful thing about a laparoscopy is that your doctor will likely be able to treat the endometriosis at the time of surgery with cautery, laser, or excision (cutting it out). Eliminating as much endometriosis as possible

in this way may relieve your pain for a considerable period of time.

Even though laparoscopy is a relatively small surgery, it's still surgery. It's still invasive and carries some minor risks. Because of this, some women choose to try various treatments first, assuming endometriosis may be the problem. Laparoscopy can always be done at a later time if you so choose.

There are limited things you can do on your own to improve endometriosis. The measures discussed in chapter 2 that may help symptoms around your period are certainly appropriate: heat, raspberry tea, ibuprofen, plenty of fluids, and fiber. If those are truly controlling your symptoms, that may be enough. But don't delay seeking medical care if you're still struggling with pain. You shouldn't be out of commission every month with your period.

Prescription-strength NSAIDs (nonsteroidal anti-inflammatory drugs) and similar medications may be very helpful. Some that are frequently used include tramadol, naproxen, and higher-dose ibuprofen. These work best when started at the first sign of pain; waiting until your period becomes excessively painful will make them less effective.

Oral contraceptives (OCPs, or birth control pills) may also work well. OCPs decrease the prostaglandins produced by the pelvic organs, which decreases the cramping and pain. These medications also work by decreasing the growth of the endometrium and the endometrial implants. There's less tissue to bleed at the time of menstruation, also leading to less pain. Using OCPs continuously can be a great option. There's no medical need to have a period every month for most women. OCPs can be taken on a schedule that will allow a period only every three months or even once a year. For many women with mild to moderate endometriosis, this may be all the treatment they need.

Continuous progestin medications may also be helpful in controlling symptoms. Options include Depo-Provera, given by injection every three months, and the levonorgestrel-containing intrauterine contraceptive device (IUD) Mirena. For women who choose an IUD, this often provides a simple and effective long-term method to control symptoms.

When these measures aren't sufficient to control symptoms, it's time for the "big guns." Oral danazol has a long history of improving pain from endometriosis. However, danazol has significant androgen (male hormone) activity, and many women experience side effects such as weight gain, oily skin, and even excess hair growth or voice changes. It's a difficult medication to use in every way and isn't prescribed much today.

Gonadotropin-releasing hormone (GnRH) agonists are at least as effective as danazol, and they don't have androgenic side effects. Remember that endometriosis needs estrogen to grow and function. Without estrogen, endometriosis "goes to sleep." These medications temporarily stop your ovaries from making estrogen, and the endometriosis stops functioning. You can think of it as a medical menopause. Most women stop having periods completely while on GnRH agonists. The most common such medication is Lupron Depot, given by injection monthly or every three months. Others include Zoladex (an implant under the skin) or Synarel (a daily nasal spray).

Because of the lack of estrogen in their system, many women using GnRH agonists experience symptoms such as hot flashes, night sweats, and vaginal dryness. A few may experience muscle and joint pain. In my experience, though, most women generally feel so much better without the pelvic pain that these side effects are only a minor inconvenience. This medication can be truly life-changing for women with severe endometriosis symptoms.

GnRH agonists can be used alone for up to six months. Because they stop estrogen production, using them longer involves too high a risk of losing bone mineral. To combat that risk and also to minimize side effects, "add-back therapy" is an option. The best-studied add-back regimen is norethindrone (5 mg daily), but there are other options as well. Add-back therapy can be started as soon as you begin GnRH agonists or any time prior to six months of use. These treatment regimens have been studied for up to two years, showing that bone mineral is usually preserved well. If you choose this option, you should also take 1,000 mg of calcium daily.

A woman with endometriosis will likely go through a series of different treatments during her reproductive life. She may be on OCPs for several years, starting soon after her periods begin, until she chooses to become pregnant. Pregnancy is wonderful for endometriosis! If a woman has difficulty conceiving because of endometriosis, treating it laparoscopically is likely to improve her ability to get pregnant. Starting OCPs relatively soon after pregnancy may delay the return of endometriosis, although we can't be absolutely certain of this.

At some point, OCPs may no longer control a woman's symptoms adequately, and she will choose a six-month course of Lupron Depot. She may have pain relief for up to a few years after treatment is completed. She may then choose to take Lupron Depot again, this time with add-back therapy for a longer period of time. That may control her symptoms well enough until she enters menopause and the endometriosis subsides.

Medication and/or conservative surgery laparoscopically doesn't adequately control symptoms in all women. A small percentage of women have endometriosis implants embedded deeply in the colon, bladder, or (rarely) other organs, necessitating more extensive surgery. Some women have a hysterectomy to try and control severe pain with periods. Unfortunately the ovaries are still present and continue to make estrogen after a hysterectomy, and about one-third of such women will require surgery again at some point. A complete hysterectomy, including removal of the ovaries, is considered definitive treatment for endometriosis, and after such surgery only about 3 percent of women will have symptoms return severe enough to require additional surgery.

Endometriosis can be a tough disease to deal with. Most women with this condition can have their symptoms controlled, but they will likely need ongoing medical treatment until the time of menopause. While the treatments discussed here are very helpful for most women, they aren't the answer for everyone. If you aren't satisfied with the medical opinion of the first doctor you see, find another one. And check out the free online endometriosis forum at www .endometriosis.org.

OVARIAN CYSTS

Many people are surprised to find out that all normal ovaries form cysts every month. The word *cyst* simply refers to a fluid collection enclosed by some type of wall. During normal ovulation, the ovary forms a cyst called a follicle around the egg cell. A normal follicle may be up to 2.5–3 cm in size (about 1 inch) when the egg is mature. As the egg is released from the ovary, the surrounding fluid is released into the pelvic cavity and is reabsorbed by the body. It's common to find one or more cysts of this type on a woman's ovaries when she has a pelvic ultrasound. And most ovaries also contain several smaller follicles a few millimeters in size. This is all normal.

Some women feel mild pain around the ovary at the time of ovulation each month. Such pain is called *mittelschmerz*. The ovary may sometimes bleed a little from the site where the egg was released, and that may cause more pain. Mittelschmerz occurs midway between two periods and usually only lasts a few hours or a day. If a little time and ibuprofen improve your symptoms, fine. If pain is persistent or more severe, birth control pills will prevent ovulation, which may help prevent new cysts from forming.

Ovaries can also form other types of cysts. An ultrasound can determine many characteristics of a cyst, including size, thickness of the wall, and whether or not there

> ### Dr. Carol Says...
>
> *"Every woman who is ovulating has an ovarian cyst every month. That's normal."*

is solid material inside the cyst. Endometriosis, for example, may form a "chocolate" cyst full of old blood from implants inside the ovary. Both benign and malignant ovarian tumors also usually show up as cysts. Many ovarian cysts cause no symptoms at all. If a cyst is seen on your pelvic ultrasound, your doctor should look for other reasons for any pain you have before deciding the cyst is to blame.

If your ovarian cyst is relatively small (less than perhaps 5 cm) and there are no other concerning findings, it's appropriate to wait a month or two and see if it resolves on its own. If you're menopausal, if the cyst is larger, or if there are other concerns, you may need surgery soon to evaluate and remove the cyst. Many times this can be done via laparoscopy. If your doctor is concerned the cyst could be malignant, more extensive surgery will likely be necessary.

Oral contraceptives (OCPs) have often been prescribed for women with ovarian cysts in hopes of helping the cyst resolve sooner. While OCPs are often an appropriate treatment to prevent new cysts from developing, there's no evidence they help a cyst already present to resolve more quickly.

PELVIC INFLAMMATORY DISEASE

Pelvic inflammatory disease (PID) is one of the more painful conditions any woman can experience. It is usually caused by a sexually transmitted organism, such as chlamydia or gonorrhea, although other organisms can also cause PID. Common symptoms include pelvic and abdominal pain, painful intercourse, bleeding after intercourse or between periods, unusual vaginal discharge, and fever.

Being sexually active with more than one partner (or having sex with someone who has had more than one partner) is the biggest risk factor for PID. If you have even the slightest concern that you may have been exposed to a sexually transmitted disease (STD), see your doctor and get tested. Gonorrhea, chlamydia, and many other STDs may cause no symptoms early on. Getting treated at that time will dramatically lessen your chances of developing PID. Chlamydia is so common that any woman under age twenty-five who is having sex should be tested every year, even if she has no symptoms.

Other risk factors for PID include douching or using an intrauterine contraceptive device (IUD) for contraception. The IUDs used today are so much safer in this regard than previous varieties, and by themselves they do not pose a significant risk for PID. But if you have an IUD in place and have sex with someone who has an STD, your risk of PID is higher than with either risk factor alone. Using a condom decreases your risk of acquiring an STD but does not eliminate the risk entirely.

If you may have PID, you need medical care right away. Waiting is dangerous. The longer any pelvic infection is present, the greater the risk of permanent damage to your reproductive organs, especially the fallopian tubes. Getting appropriate antibiotics as soon as possible is the best way to limit the chances for any such damage.

Your doctor will obtain a culture from the cervix at the top of your vagina and perform a pelvic exam. Where you feel pain during this exam will help your doctor know whether or not PID is likely. He may also perform an ultrasound, and he may order blood tests, looking for your body's general response to infection and for other STDs, such as hepatitis B, syphilis, and human immunodeficiency virus (HIV).

If the infection is detected early, you may be given oral antibiotics. Be sure to take all of them! If the infection is more advanced, you may be admitted to the hospital for intravenous antibiotics for a few days. Usually such treatment is sufficient, but occasionally the infection has progressed to the point where surgery is the only

> ### Dr. Carol Says...
>
> *"If you may have PID, don't wait! This is not a time to try and get better on your own. The longer you wait to get treatment, the greater the potential damage to your reproductive organs."*

option. Surgery may result in removal of the fallopian tubes, ovaries, and uterus. The point here is to get treated early. Don't let any infection remain untreated.

Even when PID is effectively treated, the infection may result in other complications. Scar tissue may develop in and around the fallopian tubes and ovaries, leading to an increased risk for infertility, ectopic pregnancy, future episodes of PID, or chronic pelvic pain.

You can't get an STD if you don't have sex or if you only have sex with a partner who has not had and does not have sex with anyone else. That's always the safest. Otherwise, please get medical care as soon as possible if you suspect you may have an STD or PID. You don't want the complications.

CHRONIC PELVIC PAIN

Other conditions may cause pelvic pain. Irritable bowel syndrome (IBS) is quite common and should be suspected if you have pain along with periods of constipation and/or diarrhea. Urinary tract infections (UTIs) can be especially frustrating if they are recurrent, and they may cause chronic pain. Pelvic muscle spasms are a more common cause of pain than many realize and may be treated by a physical therapist specializing in pelvic disorders.

Sometimes no diagnosis can be found to adequately explain ongoing pelvic pain. Pain is perceived by each person differently. There's no "pain meter" or blood test that can measure how much you're hurting. What feels just uncomfortable to one person may feel very painful to another. If you're hurting, it's worth taking seriously, and it's worth finding people to help you who take you seriously.

Pain is really nothing more than a message in your brain. It's how your brain interprets the signals it's getting from wherever you're hurting. That's often a very good thing, as pain can alert you to a problem you wouldn't know about any other way. It can keep you from a more serious injury or direct you to get help for some significant illness.

Pain can also be a great pretender. You may have seen the TV commercials stating that "depression hurts." And it's true. Many things may impact how your brain interprets the signals it receives, especially when it comes to pain. That's one reason people struggling with chronic pain need to pay close attention to things such as getting adequate rest, managing their stress, and choosing what they think about.

None of this means you're just imagining your pelvic pain. Far from it. But know that sometimes a doctor may find nothing wrong when he or she examines you. All the tests may come back normal, but you still hurt. Those may be the most frustrating situations of all.

Approximately one in five women has been forced to do something sexual in the past[1]—and that estimate is almost certainly low. Being violated through rape, attempted rape, or sexual abuse traumatizes a woman's body, mind, and soul as little else can. Physically, such abuse may initiate pain pathways in the nervous system that continue to function for many years, long after any physical injury has healed. Chronic pelvic and abdominal pain is quite common among women with a history of sexual abuse.[2]

If you've been affected by child abuse, domestic violence, or rape, my heart goes out to you in a very special way. You deserve to be treated with gentleness, kindness, and great respect. You survived! And the way your body has responded is no fault or choice of your own. It's not all in your head. Your body has been affected, and you deserve the very best care possible.

It may be difficult to determine which part of you needs treatment first or most. Be gentle with yourself. Seek out a gynecologist with whom you can feel safe when you're ready to have a medical evaluation. If nothing is found to be medically wrong, that reassurance itself may ease one part of your anxiety, even if it's frustrating.

I also encourage you to get help from someone skilled in abuse or trauma recovery: a therapist, a psychologist, a pastor, or an appropriate self-help group. Not every professional or pastor will be skilled in this area. Keep looking until you find someone with whom you feel safe and who has experience helping women in your situation. Addressing the mental and emotional effects of what you experienced may significantly improve your physical symptoms also.

These resources may help you find appropriate support and help:

+ RAINN (Rape, Abuse, and Incest National Network): www.rainn.org
+ National Domestic Violence Hotline: www.thehotline.org
+ National Association of Adult Survivors of Child Abuse: www.naasca.org
+ Stop It Now: www.stopitnow.org
+ National Association for Christian Recovery: www.nacr.org

This book is such a limiting place to address such a significant problem. Please know that you're not alone. And please keep searching until you find healing for the pain in both your body and your soul.

A Few Questions

Q: Will a hysterectomy cure my pelvic pain?

A: Sometimes. If your pain is caused by endometriosis, chronic pelvic inflammatory disease, uterine fibroids, or some other anatomical problem in your reproductive organs, your pain will likely be improved through a hysterectomy. But a number of women have pelvic pain without a clear anatomic reason, and a hysterectomy is not likely to improve their pain. If you are considering a hysterectomy, ask your doctor what you should realistically expect.

Q: Is pelvic congestion syndrome a cause for pelvic pain?

A: Pelvic congestion syndrome (PCS) is quite controversial. Varicose veins in the pelvis are thought to be the reason for pain in women so affected. An MRI or diagnostic venogram may help diagnose the condition. Some women find pain relief after material is injected to block the dilated veins. PCS should only be considered after you've been evaluated by a gynecologist, gastroenterologist, and general surgeon. An interventional radiologist would be the physician involved in the diagnosis and treatment of PCS.

Chapter 4

WHEN IT'S NOT NORMAL
PART 2: BLEEDING

ABNORMAL VAGINAL BLEEDING is one of the most common problems for which women visit their gynecologist. If the timing, frequency, duration, or amount of bleeding is abnormal, it can disrupt so much of your life. Approximately 10 percent of women experience abnormal uterine bleeding (AUB) at some point between the time of puberty and menopause.

Chapter 2 described normal menstrual cycles in more detail. Briefly normal menstrual bleeding happens about once a month and lasts three to seven days. Typically the heaviest bleeding occurs during the second or third day and then lightens significantly during the remaining days. On a normal heavy day, a woman may need to change a pad or tampon up to every one to two hours—but if that quantity of bleeding lasts more than several hours, it is certainly abnormal. Bleeding is also abnormal if it occurs at unpredictable times, lasts longer than seven days, or occurs at a frequency that is different from about once a month.

I still remember my mother suffering with severe bleeding, and as a physician I've helped many women with these problems. I know how frightening and frustrating this can be. So what can you do about it?

DETERMINE THE CATEGORY

There are two primary categories of AUB. The first involves various anatomical problems involving the uterus itself, such as uterine fibroids or abnormalities in the uterine lining (endometrium), and is considered *ovulatory*. The other involves abnormalities outside the uterus, such as hormonal problems or dysfunction in the blood's clotting system, and is considered *anovulatory*. Treatment for these two categories of bleeding may be quite different.

A menstrual calendar (see chapter 2) can be very helpful in determining whether or not you may be ovulating and whether your bleeding is more likely an anatomical problem or a hormone issue. If your periods are mostly monthly but are long or heavy, or if you have normal periods but also bleed at "extra" times between periods, you're probably ovulating. If your bleeding is relatively unpredictable and has no monthly pattern, you're probably not ovulating regularly.

UTERINE FIBROIDS

One common reason for AUB is uterine fibroids. Fibroids form when individual muscle cells within the uterus become independent and multiply to form a nodule or growth. They can be small (1 cm or less) or very large. I've operated on fibroids as large as a grapefruit. A woman may have a single small or large fibroid, and I've also seen cases where a woman's uterus contained more than twenty fibroids. Fibroids can develop within the uterine cavity, within the uterine wall, or on the outside of the uterus (and, more rarely, other places also).

Health Tip

Abnormal uterine bleeding fits one or more of these characteristics:

- *Does not occur approximately once a month*
- *Lasts longer than three to seven days*
- *Is excessively heavy*
- *Occurs at unpredictable times*

Fibroids are almost always benign. Many women are able to live with fibroids for years with few or no symptoms. Fibroids typically grow in response to estrogen and progesterone. They tend to show up during a woman's thirties and forties, and they often shrink or disappear after menopause. If a woman's fibroids are relatively small and are causing few symptoms, there's absolutely no reason to worry about them at all. These fibroids are not cancer, do not turn into cancer, and do not increase a woman's risk of developing cancer.

In rare cases (much less than 1 percent), uterine enlargement may be caused by leiomyosarcoma, a serious malignant disease. Unfortunately the only truly reliable way to make this diagnosis is at the time of surgical removal. Your doctor may be concerned if your uterus is extremely large, if it is growing rapidly, or if you develop symptoms after menopause. In these cases leiomyosarcoma may be more likely, and you may need surgery quickly.

But what if fibroids are causing you symptoms? Fibroids that are in or near the uterine cavity may cause heavy bleeding severe enough to require an emergency blood transfusion. Some fibroids may cause significant pelvic pain or may be large enough to put severe pressure on the rectum, bladder, or vagina. Occasionally fibroids in or near the uterine cavity may contribute to infertility or miscarriages.

If the fibroids are large enough, your doctor will be able to feel an enlarged uterus when performing a pelvic exam. A pelvic ultrasound is usually recommended to make certain of the diagnosis. Sometimes an MRI can provide further information if the ultrasound is unclear or if it is needed to plan further treatment.

There's nothing you can do to prevent fibroids. Women with a family member who had fibroids and African American women develop fibroids more frequently. That said, women who are overweight or obese tend to develop fibroids more frequently, and one study showed that women who exercise regularly develop fibroids less frequently.[1] These factors may be important because of the estrogen effect. Extra body weight increases your estrogen level, and regular exercise helps control your weight and thereby decreases your estrogen level. Less estrogen results in less stimulation for any fibroids to grow.

Over-the-counter medications such as ibuprofen or acetaminophen may help lessen the discomfort some fibroids cause during your periods. If your periods are heavy, you may need iron supplements, but don't use them for more than a few months unless you're under a doctor's care. Adequate water intake and dietary fiber will lessen the constipation that can be worse with some fibroids. Although some herbal supplements claim to help shrink fibroids, there are no reliable studies showing that to be the case. However, red raspberry and other herbal teas may help ease the discomfort fibroids may cause. Some years ago it was thought that progesterone may help shrink fibroids, but we now know that it usually doesn't help at all.

Sometimes oral contraceptives will lessen the bleeding and pain associated with fibroids, but not always. If they do help, this is a relatively inexpensive way to control your symptoms. If the fibroids are small and not distorting the uterine cavity, a progestin-containing IUD (intrauterine device) may also help decrease bleeding for some women. Ulipristal acetate (UPA) is one of the newest medication options. It works by blocking progesterone action and may decrease fibroid size significantly when used for up to three months. Studies are now being done to evaluate longer-term use.

Lupron Depot and other GnRH agonists are usually given by

injection and will temporarily shrink most fibroids significantly. They do so by blocking the ovary's production of estrogen, and therefore women taking these medications often have symptoms of menopause such as hot flashes. Fibroids will regrow to their original size shortly after a woman stops using these injections, but they may be helpful if a woman is nearing menopause or is preparing for surgery and is only likely to need them for a matter of months.

A number of newer procedures being used to treat fibroids are worth considering. If the fibroids are quite small but causing a lot of bleeding, endometrial ablation (destroying the uterine lining) may decrease the bleeding significantly. Uterine artery embolization (UAE) can block the blood supply to the fibroids using a catheter inserted through an artery in the leg, causing the fibroids to shrink. Radiofrequency during laparoscopy and MRI-guided high-energy ultrasounds are also being used to damage fibroid tissue, causing them to shrink. Any of these procedures may decrease a woman's ability to get pregnant in the future.

A myomectomy surgically removes the fibroids while leaving the uterus in place. It may be done through the cervix (hysteroscopically), through a laparoscope, or via an abdominal incision, depending on where the fibroids are located. Most women who choose to are able to conceive after a myomectomy, but a Cesarean section is usually recommended for delivery to prevent the uterine scar from tearing during labor. Additionally, 10 to 25 percent of women will need further surgery at some point after a myomectomy because of other fibroids developing.

Fibroids may return or enlarge after any of the above treatments. The only way to permanently get rid of fibroids is by doing a hysterectomy—removing the uterus. There are several ways of performing a hysterectomy: abdominal, vaginal, laparoscopic, or supracervical. Any hysterectomy will permanently eliminate the fibroids. The good news is that a woman's ovaries usually do not need to be removed in this case, so immediate menopause is not a concern. The type of hysterectomy you have is a matter to discuss with your doctor, as the size or position of the fibroids may make one or more types of hysterectomy impossible.

At the time of this writing, there is a considerable controversy over the use of morcellators to remove fibroids at the time of myomectomy or hysterectomy. Inserted through a laparoscopic incision, these devices slice the fibroids into small pieces so they can be removed without making a large abdominal incision. In a few cases, undetected leiomyosarcoma (a serious form of cancer) in the uterus has been allowed to spread more widely by the use of this procedure. This controversy is far from over, but talk with your doctor about this if you plan on laparoscopic surgery for your fibroids. My suggestion: seriously consider asking your doctor not to use a morcellator.

POLYCYSTIC OVARY SYNDROME (PCOS)

PCOS is the most common hormone abnormality in reproductive-aged women, affecting approximately one in ten women between puberty and menopause. I don't like the term *polycystic ovary syndrome* because the very small ovarian cysts aren't at all important in themselves. The hormone abnormalities are the problem.

A lot of research has been done to discover the cause of PCOS. It tends to run in families, but no one has yet discovered a specific gene causing it. This condition carries three primary features. With any two of these, you have PCOS:

1. Irregular or absent periods (not ovulating normally)

2. Excess production or activity of male hormones (androgens), such as testosterone

3. Multiple small cysts (less than 1 cm) on the ovaries

Although an ultrasound is often performed, a woman's menstrual history, physical exam, and laboratory tests are what's important in choosing treatment. The small ovarian cysts in themselves don't cause any problems. Women with PCOS have all the components necessary to ovulate: the pituitary gland can produce its hormones, the ovary can produce estrogen, eggs are present in the ovary, and the uterine lining can respond to the appropriate hormone signals by bleeding. What's missing is the normal monthly cyclic signal that controls the whole ovulation process. What we don't know is precisely what disrupts that monthly cyclic signal in most women with PCOS.

PCOS may begin soon after a girl reaches puberty and often becomes worse during her twenties. Thankfully, during a woman's later thirties and forties, the symptoms often decrease and may disappear entirely. Because women with PCOS ovulate infrequently, if at all, infertility is common. (Read more about fertility treatments that help with ovulation in chapter 7.)

But there are several other reasons to worry about PCOS even if you're not trying to get pregnant:

+ Excess hair growth (hirsutism), acne, or other skin changes
+ Excess body weight and obesity
+ Risk for endometrial hyperplasia and cancer
+ Risk for diabetes
+ Risk for cardiovascular disease

Women with PCOS are frequently overweight, though not always. The hormone changes in PCOS make it more difficult for many women to lose weight, and excess weight makes the symptoms of PCOS even worse. It's a vicious cycle. But the good news is that losing even 10 to 15 percent of your body weight may make a significant difference in all the other problems PCOS can bring, including making both conceiving and carrying a pregnancy easier. For example, if you weigh three hundred pounds, that would mean losing thirty pounds. If you're overweight and have PCOS, it's worth extraordinary effort to lose even a small amount of your extra weight.

Dr. Carol Says...

To improve or eliminate symptoms of PCOS, eliminate or decrease processed foods, especially processed carbohydrates.

PCOS involves some significant abnormalities in a woman's total-body metabolism. Two of the most important are unopposed estrogen and insulin resistance. When a woman ovulates normally, her ovaries produce progesterone between the time of ovulation and her next period. That progesterone stops the growth-inducing action of estrogen on the uterine lining (endometrium) and allows it to mature in preparation for either pregnancy or menstruation. As I've said before, no ovulation, no progesterone—and the uterine lining keeps on growing. That unchecked growth can lead to unpredictable bleeding (not a true period) and eventually hyperplasia (abnormal overgrowth) and/or cancer.

Most women with PCOS have insulin resistance. This means it takes a lot more insulin for their body's cells to metabolize blood sugar than it does for someone else. Over time, their body's ability to produce enough insulin may become overwhelmed, and diabetes may develop. That is an oversimplified explanation, but it helps describe why so many women with PCOS develop type 2 diabetes. Some researchers have thought this insulin resistance may be the underlying cause of all cases of PCOS, but that hasn't turned out to be the case.

Whether because of obesity, insulin resistance, or other factors, women with PCOS have an increased risk of hypertension (high blood pressure), lipid abnormalities (high cholesterol), metabolic syndrome (a combination of these risk factors), and cardiovascular disease. Does all that sound pretty serious? We may not know the specific cause of PCOS, but we know enough about it to effectively manage the problems it brings. Dealing with it early can give you a good chance of preventing problems in the future.

What can you do on your own? By far, the single most important thing you can do is manage your weight. Exercise is helpful, but the hormone changes in PCOS make it almost impossible for many women to lose weight without significantly changing their diet. Some women can completely reverse the symptoms of PCOS simply through dietary changes.

To understand how to lose weight when you have PCOS, you must remember how important insulin resistance is in this condition. Decrease your insulin level, and many of the symptoms of PCOS get better. And what stimulates insulin? Blood sugar. Glucose. It's as simple as that. Any diet that decreases blood sugar will improve insulin resistance, improve PCOS symptoms, and help you lose weight.

The Mediterranean diet has the best track record for decreasing your risk for diabetes, heart disease, and stroke, even in people who already have risk factors. I tell all my patients with PCOS that the single most important dietary change they can make is decreasing or eliminating processed food. Refined grains, such as breads, pastas, cereals, and baked goods, raise blood sugar quickly. That increases insulin and worsens PCOS.

What should you eat? Important principles of the Mediterranean diet include focusing on unprocessed protein (like fish and poultry), fruits, and vegetables. There's a lot of research to recommend olive oil as well. Experts disagree about how dairy products and whole grains affect the symptoms of PCOS. I recommend modest amounts of whole grains, such as oats, brown rice, or barley. If you can't make any other changes, increase how many vegetables you eat. The increased fiber helps you feel fuller and decreases your cholesterol and blood sugar levels as well.

Inositol has been shown effective in moderating insulin levels, improving ovulation rates, and improving the hormone abnormalities of PCOS. Myoinositol (2–4 grams per day) and d-chiro-inositol (50–100 mg per day) are both helpful. You can find generic forms at most nutrition stores, or purchase Pregnitude at www.pregnitude.com or Chiral Balance at www.chiralbalance.com. (I have no opinion on these companies as a whole, only these two products.)

If your periods are irregular, it's important to have a medical evaluation for PCOS. Blood tests can confirm the diagnosis, rule out other similar conditions, and evaluate for complications such as diabetes. If you're over thirty and have had irregular periods for some time, it's likely your doctor will recommend an endometrial biopsy to rule out hyperplasia or endometrial cancer. An ultrasound may be helpful to rule out other causes of irregular bleeding.

Health Tip

Blood tests useful in PCOS:

- *Fasting blood glucose*
- *Fasting insulin*
- *Fasting lipid profile*
- *Hemoglobin A1c*
- *TSH (thyroid stimulating hormone)*
- *Prolactin*
- *DHEA-S (dehydroepiandrosterone sulfate)*
- *Testosterone (total and free)*
- *FSH (follicle stimulating hormone)*
- *LH (luteinizing hormone)*
- *AMH (anti-mullerian hormone)*
- *Consider glucose tolerance test*

Birth control pills do two things well for women with PCOS: they control irregular periods (thereby also preventing endometrial cancer) and decrease excess testosterone production from the ovaries. Spironolactone (100 mg per day) blocks the action of testosterone on your skin's hair follicles and may decrease excess hair growth when used regularly for a few months. Using these two medications together has been a mainstay of PCOS treatment for years. Of course, neither of these medications can be used if you're trying to get pregnant.

More recently metformin (1,500–2,000 mg per day) has been used quite successfully for PCOS. It targets insulin resistance, resulting in lower insulin levels, lower blood sugar (if high), lower androgen levels, and often improved ovulation. Many women find they can lose weight easier while taking metformin. It is probably the best medication treatment available to decrease the long-term risks of PCOS, including diabetes and cardio-vascular disease. Metformin can be used with birth control pills and/or spironolactone if needed, and it can be used alone or with fertility medications if you're trying to get pregnant. Some women have gas-trointestinal side effects with metformin, such as cramping, gas, or diarrhea, which are often temporary. Increasing your dose gradually may give your GI system the necessary time to adjust.

Lastly, laparoscopic ovarian drilling has been used in women with PCOS for many years. Laser, cautery, or other methods are used to make multiple small openings in the capsule (covering) of the ovary. This improves ovulation rates and decreases androgen production in many cases. However, the risks of surgery and the likelihood of symptoms recurring later make surgery less attractive than lifestyle and medication management.

If you struggle with PCOS, I encourage you to work hard on developing a healthy eating plan that you can continue long-term and to control your weight. PCOS may make you feel like your body has failed you. *You* take charge. Become the master of your metabolism. Don't remain a victim of PCOS.

OTHER CONDITIONS

Blood-clotting problems. Up to 20 percent of women with abnormal uterine bleeding have an abnormality in the blood-clot-ting system. This is especially important when periods are excessively heavy right from the time of puberty. These genetic disorders may also show up as frequent or easy bruising or nosebleeds or bleeding after dental work or minor surgery. Other family members may also have bleeding problems. Special blood tests are required to evaluate the proteins in your blood that are responsible for normal clotting. If you're concerned, talk with your doctor about blood tests to evaluate your blood-clotting system.

Endometrial polyp. The uterine lining (endometrium) may develop fingerlike projections of tissue that can bleed abnormally and do not slough off during normal menstruation. An ultrasound may indicate a polyp is likely. Hysteroscopy either in the office or in the operating room can allow your doctor to both see the polyp and usually remove it completely. A pathology report will indicate whether the polyp is atypical, indicating an increased risk of uterine cancer in the future.

Thyroid disease. Hypothyroidism (inadequate production of thyroid hormone) affects about 10 percent of women at some point during their lives, and AUB is one possible symptom. Other possible symptoms include weight gain, dry skin and hair, fatigue, constipation, depression, and others. If hypothyroidism is the cause of your AUB, appropriate thyroid hormone replacement should improve your bleeding.

AUB at puberty. During the first several years a young woman has periods, she may not ovulate regularly. This may lead to heavy and irregular periods. If her blood-clotting system is normal (see above), it may just be a matter of time; cycles may become normal within a few years. Birth control pills, taken for a while, may be the best way to control the heavy irregular bleeding.

AUB near menopause. During the last few years prior to menopause, a woman usually ovulates less and less frequently. Her reproductive hormones (especially estrogen) go through increasingly dramatic changes, which often result in heavier or irregular bleeding. There's also an increasing likelihood of other problems including fibroids or endometrial polyps. An endometrial biopsy and pelvic ultrasound are usually needed. If those tests are normal, medications or endometrial ablation may be needed to control bleeding until periods stop with menopause.

OTHER TREATMENTS

Whatever the cause of AUB, and especially if no specific cause is discovered, some treatment options are often helpful for decreasing heavy abnormal uterine bleeding.

Among their effects, birth control pills decrease the growth of the endometrium. With less tissue to bleed, menstrual periods are usually lighter and less painful. Good low-dose options are now available, allowing many women to use birth control pills safely who could not use older, higher-dose pills. If you don't smoke and don't have other medical risk factors, you might be able to take low-dose birth control pills all the way until menopause.

Tranexamic acid (Lysteda) is a nonhormonal medication that can be taken for up to five days each month by women with heavy but ovulatory menstrual cycles. It should not be used at the same time as hormonal contraception (pills, patches, rings, etc.). In most women the risks are very low, and menstrual bleeding may be much less.

Endometrial ablation removes much of the uterine lining through freezing, cautery, heat destruction, or surgical removal. Most women who choose this treatment are very satisfied with the results, and up to 60 percent of women have no periods at all after ablation. However, up to 30 percent of women who have this procedure prior to age forty-five will develop AUB again before menopause.

A levonorgestrel-releasing intrauterine contraceptive device (Mirena, Skyla) is as good at controlling AUB as endometrial ablation, and it's reversible. The device is inserted into the uterine cavity in a simple office procedure and is effective for up to five years. (See more about IUDs in chapter 5.)

The definitive treatment for abnormal uterine bleeding is, of course, hysterectomy, even if no specific cause is identified for your AUB. Once the uterus is removed, there's nothing there to bleed! And many hysterectomies are still being done for heavy bleeding when no other treatment has been successful. While hysterectomy should not be the first choice, or even the second or third choice, sometimes it becomes the best option.

There are almost always several treatment options available to manage your abnormal uterine bleeding. Think through what's important to you, and talk about the different options with your doctor. You may have to try more than one option before you find what works best for you.

And remember that God understands what you're going through. When Jesus was here on Earth, a woman who had been bleeding for twelve years came to Him for help. He graciously healed her, and she was grateful. (See Luke 8:43–48.) He will be gracious with you too.

A FEW QUESTIONS

Q: Can any supplements decrease my abnormal bleeding?

A: A number of supplements have been recommended for this issue. Unfortunately there are no good quality studies demonstrating their effectiveness.

Q: Will exercise or a specific diet help my uterine fibroids?

A: As mentioned in this chapter, one study demonstrated that women who exercise regularly had a lower risk of fibroids. It would be logical to conclude that a regular exercise program and healthy diet that helps you attain an ideal weight would slow down the growth of fibroids, but there is no research yet to prove this.

Q: Does stress make PCOS worse?

A: Some women's reproductive systems are very sensitive to periods of stress. Managing stress well through adequate rest, appropriate exercise, and supportive friends may help you ovulate more easily and manage your weight better. These factors may improve other symptoms of PCOS as well.

Chapter 5

CONTRACEPTION

I WILL ALWAYS REMEMBER a heartrending story one of my professors told us when I was in medical school. A young woman in a third-world country already had four children. She knew the financial and physical pressures more children would bring but had no means of contraception available. Each month she spent a lot of time finding any excuse possible to avoid sleeping with her husband and then praying for her period to come.

There's no question that relatively safe and effective contraception has brought many benefits to many women. But it has also brought some difficult decisions and ethical challenges that were unheard of just a few years ago. The Affordable Care Act has brought some of these challenges to the forefront in a new way.

There's one thing I know for sure: if you don't have sex, you won't get pregnant. I've cared for many women who became pregnant while using various forms of contraception. (I've cared for many more women who became pregnant while not using any contraception at all!) No birth control method is perfect. Some methods are riskier for your health than others, and some have other potential health benefits beyond preventing pregnancy. It's likely you will find one or more that will meet your needs.

And then there's the important question some women of faith wonder about: *Should* I use birth control? Near the end of this chapter, we'll address that question specifically.

PRINCIPLES OF CONTRACEPTION

There are so many contraceptive choices available today that it helps to take a step back and look at the big picture. For a woman to become pregnant, several things must happen. A healthy, mature egg must be released from the ovary at the right time. Healthy sperm must be present in a woman's reproductive tract at that same time. The egg and sperm must find each other, which normally happens in the fallopian tube. The early embryo must find its way into the uterine cavity and must attach to a mature, receptive uterine wall. The hormonal environment must be supportive of the early embryo's development.

Different methods of contraception focus on disrupting this process at any of the points along the way. Some methods block the process of ovulation, preventing a mature egg from developing and releasing from the ovary. Some methods keep sperm from entering the woman's reproductive tract. Some methods keep sperm and egg from coming in contact with each other. Some methods affect the ability of the embryo to attach to the uterine wall and begin development. For some people these differences are very important. Unfortunately there is no method currently available to prevent men from making healthy sperm. (It's very sad that men are left out of this equation as much as they are!)

Other aspects of contraception are also important. Some are much more effective at preventing pregnancy than others. Some have additional health benefits beyond preventing pregnancy. Some require you to do something each time you have intercourse. Some require your action each day or possibly each week or each month. Some are effective for years at a time. Most are reversible, while a few are permanent.

These are the factors women, their partners, and their doctors consider every day when making contraceptive choices. The following table presents a brief overview of most currently available contraceptive methods. Keep in mind that the risks and other health benefits may or may not apply to you; these especially need to be discussed with your doctor. Reversible methods are listed first, starting with the most effective. Irreversible methods are listed last.

Method	When you need to take action	Effectiveness at preventing pregnancy	Other potential health benefits	Possible health risks	Primary method of action
Copper T IUD (Paragard)	Every ten years	Excellent	None	Heavier periods	Limits egg and sperm movement
Progestin IUD (Mirena, Skyla)	Every three to five years	Excellent	Decreased pain and bleeding	Minimal	Prevents ovulation

Method	When you need to take action	Effectiveness at preventing pregnancy	Other potential health benefits	Possible health risks	Primary method of action
Hormone implant	Every three years	Excellent	Possibly decreased bleeding	Minimal	Prevents ovulation
Hormone injections	Every three months	Very good	Possibly decreased bleeding	Weight gain	Prevents ovulation
Combined oral contraceptive pills (OCPs)	Daily	Very good if used as directed	Decrease in pain, bleeding, ovarian cysts, and risk of some cancers	Unsafe for smokers over age thirty-five or those with certain health problems	Prevents ovulation
Progestin-only pill (minipill)	Daily, at the same time	Good if used as directed	Safe while breast-feeding	Some have irregular bleeding	Prevents ovulation
Hormone patch	Each week for three weeks each month	Good (if under 198 pounds)	Similar to OCPs	Similar to OCPs	Prevents ovulation
Vaginal ring	Monthly to insert and remove	Very good if used as directed	Similar to OCPs	Similar to OCPs	Prevents ovulation
Plan B and similar emergency contraception	Within seventy-two hours of intercourse	Fair	None	May lead to irregular bleeding	Controversial: may prevent ovulation and embryo implantation

Method	When you need to take action	Effectiveness at preventing pregnancy	Other potential health benefits	Possible health risks	Primary method of action
Ella emergency contraception	Within five days of intercourse	Fair	None	May lead to delayed period	Prevents ovulation and embryo implantation
Diaphragm or cervical cap	Each act of intercourse	Fair	None significant	Vaginal irritation	Prevents sperm entry
Male condom	Each act of intercourse	Fair	Decreases risk of STDs	None significant	Prevents sperm entry
Female condom	Each act of intercourse	Fair	Decreases risk of STDs	None significant	Prevents sperm entry
Spermicide	Each act of intercourse	Poor	Some may decrease risk of STDs	Vaginal irritation	Prevents sperm entry
Natural family planning	Daily planning	Fair to good (depends on couple)	Knowledge of personal cycles	None	Requires refraining from intercourse during fertile period
Male sterilization (vasectomy)	One time	Excellent (irreversible)	None significant	Negligible	Prevents sperm entry entirely
Tubal ligation ("tying tubes")	One time	Excellent (irreversible)	May decrease risk of ovarian cancer	Requires surgery	Prevents sperm/egg fertilization

Method	When you need to take action	Effective- ness at preventing pregnancy	Other potential health benefits	Possible health risks	Primary method of action
Transcer- vical tubal ligation (Essure)	One time	Excellent (irrevers- ible)	Unclear	Possibly increased pain and bleeding	Prevents sperm/ egg fertil- ization

Now for some specifics about each of the primary methods of contraception.

IUDS AND HORMONAL IMPLANTS

Intrauterine contraceptive devices (IUDs) have been around a long time and have gone through many variations. A few decades ago, they got a bad reputation for causing pelvic infections, including PID (pelvic inflammatory disease) and infertility. Significant design changes in currently available IUDs have mostly eliminated these risks. However, someone who has multiple sexual partners and is therefore at a higher risk of STDs should probably not use an IUD, since doing so may increase her risk of a significant pelvic infection if she does develop an STD. IUDs don't decrease your risk of con- tracting a sexually transmitted disease.

An IUD is placed inside your uterus by your doctor in a simple outpatient procedure. Most women find the IUD placement to be only mildly uncomfortable. The IUD is immediately effective in pre- venting pregnancy (as long as you're not already pregnant).

The progestin-containing IUDs can also decrease how much bleeding you have with your periods, and some women stop having periods entirely. This is often an effective treatment for heavy and painful menstrual periods. These IUDs are effective for three to five years, depending on which brand is used. The copper-containing IUD is effective for up to ten years. With this IUD, periods generally remain regular but may also be more painful and heavier.

The hormonal implant is placed under the skin of your arm in a simple outpatient procedure under local anesthesia and lasts for at least three years. It is considered, statistically, one of the most effec- tive methods of contraception available. Most women don't ovulate while using the implant and therefore don't have periods. While the IUDs can usually be removed simply by pulling on the attached string, removing the implant involves a small incision under local anesthesia.

Fertility usually returns quickly after one of these devices is removed, certainly within one menstrual cycle. The risk of long-term health problems is minimal with any of these methods.

Many Christians are concerned about the way in which IUDs prevent pregnancy. The primary method by which the copper-containing IUD does so is by creating an inhospitable environment for eggs and sperm. The fallopian tube does not move as effectively, and the fluid inside the fallopian tube becomes hostile to the egg. The cervical mucus becomes toxic to sperm and difficult for the sperm to pass through. Eggs and sperm do not have the chance to reach each other most of the time.

Health Tip

Consider a progestin IUD if:

• *You want long-acting, reversible contraception*

• *You want to lessen heavy periods*

• *You aren't sexually active with multiple partners*

• *You're willing to accept the very small risk of ovulation, fertilization, and disruption of an early embryo*

The primary method by which progestin-containing IUDs and the hormonal implant prevent pregnancy is by preventing ovulation. The progestin hormone suppresses egg development, as evidenced by how often the women using these methods stop having periods. The fallopian tubes also move less effectively, and the cervical mucus becomes hostile to sperm.

However, with any IUD, an egg and sperm may come together and fertilization may occur. No reliable data exists to prove exactly how frequently this occurs in women using IUDs. Fertilization would definitely occur more often with the copper-containing IUD, since it doesn't interfere with ovulation. Evidence that the copper-containing IUD probably also interferes with implantation is the fact that it's also an effective "emergency contraceptive," preventing pregnancy when inserted soon after unplanned or unwanted intercourse.

If this debate doesn't matter to you, these so-called LARCs (long-acting reversible contraceptives) are very effective at preventing pregnancy and can be a good choice for many women, from a health perspective.

If this debate does matter to you and you don't want to do anything to possibly disrupt the implantation of an early embryo, the copper-containing IUD would not be a good choice for you. Because the progestin-containing IUDs generally prevent ovulation, the chance of disrupting implantation would be much less, and some people would consider this an appropriate option. But there are certainly other effective options available for most women if you want to stay away from this controversial area entirely.

HORMONE INJECTIONS

Depo-Provera is the only contraceptive injection available in the United States, though others are available in some other countries. The injection every three months effectively prevents ovulation most of the time. Almost all women using these injections will have a change in their menstrual pattern, and many stop having periods entirely.

Additionally Depo-Provera can remain in your body for quite a long time. Injections need to be given every three months to reliably prevent pregnancy, but it may take up to nine months or longer for normal fertility to return once you stop the injections.

Depo-Provera can also be an effective treatment for some women with endometriosis or painful, heavy periods. However, if heavy or irregular bleeding is your primary problem, this isn't a good option, as the injections cause some women to develop irregular or prolonged bleeding when they didn't have that problem before. Weight gain is common, though usually no more than five to ten pounds. Some gain much more than that, and weight gain is one of the primary reasons more women don't choose this method.

There is some concern that long-term use of Depo-Provera may result in loss of bone mineral in otherwise healthy young women. Fortunately the lost bone mineral is usually regained once women stop using the injections, though it may take a few years. For this reason, many doctors recommend limiting Depo-Provera use to two years and taking calcium (1,000 mg daily) during this time. This loss of bone mineral may be especially concerning for adolescents at a time when they should be rapidly gaining bone mineral. While Depo-Provera can be an effective and simple method for adolescents to use for contraception, it may be best to only consider this option for young women for whom other methods are not a realistic choice.

ORAL CONTRACEPTIVE PILLS (OCPs)

Some would argue that the development of the pill was a significant trigger in the sexual revolution of the 1960s. Few medications have been better studied than combined oral contraceptives (OCPs). They're called *combined* because all "normal" OCPs contain both a synthetic estrogen and a synthetic progestin. There are many varieties, doses, and packaging variations, most with differences in the type of progestin used. These variations have been developed to try to find the lowest possible dose that will reliably prevent ovulation while giving the fewest side effects.

Please note: Almost everything in this section applies just as much to the contraceptive skin patch and the vaginal ring. All three methods provide the same hormones through various routes in order to prevent ovulation. The differences are minor, and the hormones involved are basically the same.

Health Tip

Consider oral contraceptives if:

- *You need to control irregular periods*
- *You're willing to take a pill every day*
- *You don't smoke*
- *You want to lessen acne or excess body hair*
- *You're concerned about endometriosis*
- *You want to decrease your risk of ovarian cancer*

As the doses of hormones used in OCPs have decreased, so have most of the side effects. But the risk of breakthrough ovulation has also increased a little. As a result, the lowest-dose pills have a slightly increased risk of "failure" (becoming pregnant on the pill) and of breakthrough bleeding.

We don't have space to discuss the dozens of different brands of OCPs and the many generics available. Even the best doctor may not be able to recommend the best pill for you on the first try. It may be partly a matter of trial and error. Tell your doctor what's important to you besides not getting pregnant, such as limiting weight gain, improving acne, or decreasing pain with your periods. Together you will choose a pill to try for a couple months. Unless you have a problem that is unexpected or severe, keep taking your pills as directed for at least two cycles, and then try a different brand if you're not satisfied.

What are some of those side effects? Irregular spotting or bleeding between periods is the most common. This will often improve once your body gets into the rhythm of what to expect with the pills. If not, trying a different brand may make a big difference. Headaches, nausea, or breast tenderness are also relatively common and often temporary.

More serious side effects are rare and include blood clots in the legs or elsewhere, chest pain, severe headaches, numbness or tingling in the hands or feet, or changes in vision. Women with an increased risk of these problems, including those who smoke and are over thirty-five or who have certain medical problems, should not use OCPs.

Many women choose to use OCPs for the additional health benefits they provide besides contraception. OCPs often improve painful or heavy periods, irregular periods, and the symptoms of endometriosis. Excess hair growth (hirsutism) and acne are often improved with certain OCPs. Women who use OCPs also have a lower risk of ovarian cysts, anemia, and uterine or ovarian cancer in the future.

If you've chosen to try OCPs, how well you do on them is partly dependent on your ability to take them regularly. Place your pill pack near something you already see every day, such as your toothbrush. Take them at the same time as another medication you take daily. Or put a reminder on your smartphone. If you miss one pill, take it as soon as you can. If you miss two or more, still make up your missed pills but know that you may have an increased risk of pregnancy or irregular bleeding.

One convenient aspect of OCPs is that you can use them to schedule your period. There's no medical need to have a period every four weeks. Some women do better using OCPs continuously and scheduling periods every three months or even every year. You can also adjust your pill schedule to avoid having your period on vacation or on your wedding day. Talk with your doctor about the best way to create an appropriate schedule for you.

EMERGENCY CONTRACEPTION

Unplanned, unwanted, or unprotected intercourse may result in pregnancy if you haven't yet ovulated in your current cycle. Sperm can live for at least five days in a woman's reproductive tract and still be capable of fertilizing an egg. An egg must be fertilized within twenty-four hours after ovulation, so if you ovulated more than twenty-four hours before having intercourse, there's no chance you will become pregnant. Since most women don't know exactly when they ovulate, emergency contraception has been suggested for use anytime during a woman's cycle.

Ella (ulipristal acetate) is a form of emergency contraception that is only available by prescription. It blocks the action of progesterone and, in doing so, may delay ovulation, perhaps even by a few days. It also affects the endometrium (uterine lining) and may interfere with implantation of an embryo. It is probably most effective when taken shortly before the time of ovulation.

The other emergency contraceptives (Plan B and others) are progestin-only, and many are available without a prescription. There is much debate as to how these medications decrease the chance of pregnancy. Taken before ovulation, they may decrease the likelihood of a healthy egg being released. They also definitely affect the endometrium and may interfere with embryo implantation.

All emergency contraceptive pills currently available have only a fair chance of preventing pregnancy and are far from perfect in this regard. As with our previous discussion of IUDs, there's at least some possibility that using emergency contraception will prevent a fertilized embryo from implanting in the uterus. If that debate matters to you, don't use emergency contraception.

Barrier Methods

Condoms (female and male), diaphragms, and spermicides all must be used with each act of intercourse to be effective. It's not that hard to imagine that for the "typical user," these methods have a relatively high failure rate. That's because they may be used only part of the time, because condoms can break, and because spermicide only kills some sperm (perhaps most, but not all).

Using condoms regularly will decrease your chances of contracting a sexually transmitted disease. The important word is *decrease*, not *prevent*. I've seen too many women come for treatment of an STD when they thought they were being careful. Let me encourage you to not rely on being careful.

Natural Family Planning

Natural family planning has been used effectively by many couples for generations. If you are or grew up Catholic, you undoubtedly have heard much about this as the only contraceptive method sanctioned by the Catholic Church. The method relies on abstaining from intercourse during the period of a woman's cycle when she may become pregnant.

The principles of this method are not hard to understand. Sperm can live in a woman's reproductive tract for at least five days. The egg must be fertilized within twenty-four hours of ovulation, or pregnancy will not occur. Abstaining from intercourse from six to seven days before ovulation until after the egg is no longer viable prevents sperm from being present when an egg can be fertilized—and pregnancy cannot occur.

Challenges come when both partners aren't fully committed to this method of contraception. It won't work if, like in the story opening this chapter, you have to find creative ways to avoid your husband for a week or two every month. Both husband and wife must work together to make this method effective.

To know when to abstain, you'll need to know when you're going to ovulate. That means keeping track of your menstrual cycles religiously. If your cycles are predictable, you'll know when you are going to ovulate: about fourteen days prior to your next period. If your cycles are regular, this method can be more

Health Tip

Consider natural family planning if:

- *Your periods are relatively regular*
- *You and your husband are both committed to it*
- *You're willing to abstain from intercourse during certain times*
- *You don't want to use any hormones or barrier methods*
- *You're willing to accept a "surprise" as God's gift*

than 95 percent effective in preventing pregnancy. Unfortunately this method is more difficult to use effectively if your cycles aren't regular.

There are several resources that may help you learn this method. Some Catholic organizations offer training for couples in natural family planning. You can find helpful resources from Natural Family Planning International at www.nfpandmore.org. Or try the CycleBeads, myNFP, or other similar apps on your smartphone.

I know couples who have used natural family planning successfully for decades without any surprise pregnancies. There are also many couples who have experienced "surprises." Predicting ovulation in advance is not 100 percent accurate, and only God knows how long any given sperm cell will truly remain alive. If you choose this method, do so as a couple and with the spiritual commitment to accept any "surprise" as a blessing from God. (But isn't that the case with any contraceptive method? None is 100 percent guaranteed.)

STERILIZATION

Approximately one-third of couples choose permanent sterilization—meaning vasectomy or tubal ligation—as their method of birth control. From the perspective of health risks and costs, vasectomy is one of the least expensive and least risky ways to prevent pregnancy. Failure rates are extremely low. Some men, however, feel as though a vasectomy is an affront to their manhood. If your husband is interested, vasectomy is a wonderful option. If not, don't risk the aggravation of a marital fight.

Alternatively blocking a woman's fallopian tubes through tubal ligation can be done in several ways. When it is done at the time of a Cesarean section, there are no significant additional risks. When it is done via laparoscopy, there are the small risks of surgery. When done through the cervix (with the Essure procedure), it's important to complete the follow-up test three months later to be certain that scar tissue has completely blocked the fallopian tubes. Recent reports indicate the rate of complications such as bleeding or pain after Essure, though small, may be higher than scientists first thought.[1]

Any tubal ligation carries approximately 0.5 percent chance of "failure," meaning a pregnancy occurring in the future. (That number varies slightly depending on how the tubal ligation was done.) If a pregnancy does occur, it's more likely it will implant outside the uterus, usually in the fallopian tube (an ectopic pregnancy). If you ever suspect you may be pregnant after having a tubal ligation, get medical care right away.

Health Tip

Consider sterilization if:

- *You've had all the children you desire*
- *You don't want to worry about contraception in the future*
- *You're willing to undergo the procedure*

All of these sterilization procedures are considered permanent. Surgery to reverse a vasectomy or tubal ligation can sometimes be accomplished, but the chance of successful pregnancy is always less than before. Reversal is often expensive and involves more risks than the original procedure. If you are in any way concerned that you may regret your decision in the future, don't undergo a sterilization procedure in the first place.

SHOULD YOU USE CONTRACEPTION?

Whether or not to use contraception—and what method to use—is a big decision each couple must make for themselves. There are many factors to consider: convenience, cost, your health status, your moral/ethical values, and how it will affect your relationship.

You probably hear many voices telling you what to think. On one hand, much of modern society says any contraception is good, sex is a right, and pregnancy is an imposition on a woman's body that should be avoided unless she chooses otherwise. On the other side, one might point to the Catholic Church's position that contraception is wrong because God intended sex and procreation to be always connected and that sex without the possibility of procreation is against God's plan.

I see in Scripture that God values the unity-building aspects of sex just as much as the procreative aspects. In places such as Hebrews 13:4 and the whole Book of Song of Solomon, God celebrates the bonding between husband and wife that happens with sexual intimacy. I believe God can bless a couple that chooses to use contraception to plan their family. I have prescribed many, though definitely not all, of the contraceptive methods discussed in this chapter.

With the information provided here and with prayer, I believe you'll be able to make a contraception decision that's right for you and consistent with your faith.

A FEW QUESTIONS

Q: You haven't mentioned abortion. Why not?

A: I believe every human life is a gift from God right from its earliest moments. However, there is not adequate space in this book to do justice to such a politically and emotionally charged subject. If you're wrestling with how to handle an unwanted pregnancy or are carrying shame after having an abortion in the past, I encourage you to seek out a pregnancy resource center in your area. Other women have faced similar challenges and want to help you.

Chapter 6

YOUR HEALTHY PREGNANCY

THERE'S NOTHING LIKE the thrill of seeing a new life come into the world. That first cry. The wonder with which the new parents check out nose, fingers, and toes. Grabbing a cell-phone picture of the first time the baby is weighed. It's often magic, miracle, amazement, and instant love all at once.

Much of the time those birth moments are wonderful. Mommy and Daddy are excited. The birth may be difficult, but the joy of welcoming a new baby soon relegates the pain to just a memory. A happy family begins the journey of helping a new human being prepare for an uncertain but hopeful future.

Some birth moments, however, are tragic. I've delivered babies with serious birth defects; babies who didn't survive; and babies born far too soon who would experience months, even years, of hospitalization, pain, disability, and struggle. I've cared for mothers who experienced serious injury during birth or whose medical complications nearly resulted in their new babies being motherless. I've tried to help bring hope to mothers who had no family support or who were overwhelmed with depression or other challenges.

I want your birth experience to be wonderful. No one can guarantee a perfect baby, but there's a lot you can do to make a healthy pregnancy and a healthy baby more likely.

PLANNING FOR PREGNANCY

Preparing for parenthood is a big responsibility—physically, emotionally, financially, and spiritually. Your physical health before conceiving will affect your pregnancy and the health of your baby for years to come. Science discovers more all the time about how important preconception health can be.

Most people know that smoking and pregnancy don't go together. Smoking is harmful to a woman's eggs. Women who smoke have eggs that are older than their biological age, have a higher chance of infertility, and go through menopause earlier. Smoking during pregnancy increases the risk of problems, including miscarriage, low birth weight, preterm delivery, birth defects, and even stillbirth. I know how hard it can be to quit smoking; I watched my husband struggle to quit after smoking for forty-five years. If he can do it, you can do it too! (See Appendix B for more on this.)

Other substances may impact your fertility and pregnancy. Alcohol is a no-no. If you're going to drink and you're trying to get pregnant, it's best to avoid alcohol between ovulation and your next menstrual period—the time period when conception is going to occur. Marijuana and other recreational drugs are all detrimental. If you struggle with an addiction, the best time to get help and get clean is before you get pregnant.

Caffeine use during pregnancy is somewhat controversial. Drinking moderate amounts of coffee or tea (one to two cups per day) is probably OK while trying to conceive or during pregnancy. Heavy use (three to five cups or more per day) may decrease your fertility and affect the health of your pregnancy.

Dr. Carol Says . . .

"Making necessary changes before you get pregnant, such as quitting smoking, overcoming an addiction, and losing weight, will make for an easier and healthier pregnancy and a healthier child for decades to come."

Now comes one of the most sensitive areas we need to talk about: your weight. With two-thirds of adults in the United States being overweight or obese, we've learned a lot about how excess weight affects pregnancy. And it's not a pretty picture. Being overweight increases the chances of infertility and risks for complications during pregnancy, such as high blood pressure, preeclampsia (toxemia), diabetes, birth defects, Cesarean section, stillbirth, and more.

Maternal obesity increases the risk of both low birth weight and high birth weight. The risk of high birth weight is increased even more if the mother develops gestational diabetes (diabetes during pregnancy). High-birth-weight babies have an increased risk of injury during birth and increased risk of blood-sugar problems during the first days of life. Low birth weight can occur because the placenta's development may be stunted by maternal obesity. Babies born to overweight or obese mothers have more growth problems during childhood, either being too small or too big. They have a higher chance of childhood and adult obesity and of developing heart disease or diabetes in the future. A mother's excess body weight leads to genetic imprinting in her offspring—changes in the baby's DNA that affect that child's health throughout his or her life.[1]

Now, have I scared you enough? Yes, it's not a pretty picture. But it's not meant to be discouraging; it's meant to be motivating. Losing weight is incredibly tough for many people. You need a big enough *why* to make the extraordinary lifestyle changes that will likely be necessary and to stick with them over a long period of time. Perhaps understanding how your weight may impact your pregnancy and your hoped-for child for the rest of his or her life will be that *why* for you.

Losing even some of your excess weight before you become pregnant is one of the healthiest things you can do for you and your baby. I tell my infertility patients that losing even 10 to 15 percent of their body weight will improve their chances for getting pregnant and make for an easier pregnancy and a healthier baby. (See chapter 10 for more on managing your weight.)

Checklist for Your Preconception Doctor's Visit

- *Review your medical and pregnancy history.*
- *Evaluate any medications you use for safety in pregnancy.*
- *Review your family history for genetic illnesses.*
- *Discuss weight, diet, and lifestyle issues.*
- *PAP and STD testing, if necessary.*
- *Discuss rubella vaccine.*
- *Begin prenatal vitamins and folic acid.*
- *Review any exposure to toxins at home or work.*

Medication use during pregnancy can be a challenging topic for both patients and doctors—and herbal supplements can be just as problematic. The short answer: don't use any supplement, over-the-counter medication, or prescription while trying to conceive or during pregnancy unless you discuss it with your doctor. Medications used to treat high blood pressure, seizures, and diabetes are especially troublesome. If you're on any long-term medication, have a consultation with your obstetrician before trying to get pregnant; if necessary, medications can often be changed to ones that are safer during pregnancy.

Here are a few other useful items to think about while planning for parenthood:

+ **Get as much of your family medical history as possible.**
  This may alert you and your doctor to your risk for having a
  child with a possible genetic illness.

+ **Develop a healthy exercise program and healthy eating
  habits.** See the nutrition and exercise sections below for
  more information.

+ **Begin taking prenatal vitamins.** Taking a daily multivitamin containing at least 0.4 mg of folic acid for weeks to
  months prior to conceiving can help prevent birth defects
  affecting your baby's brain and spinal cord, preterm delivery,
  and more.

+ **Put kitty outdoors.** Cats, especially their litter boxes, may
  transmit toxoplasmosis, which can be detrimental to a developing embryo. Pregnant women should not ever clean litter
  boxes.

+ **Consider the rubella vaccine.** Rubella can lead to life-
  threatening problems for a developing embryo, including
  congenital heart disease, deafness, and more. If you're not
  immune already, seriously consider getting vaccinated.

+ **Begin tracking your menstrual cycle.** It will help you know
  when you're ovulating and help maximize your chances for
  getting pregnant soon.

+ **Get a Pap test and get screened for any STDs.** If you haven't
  received a Pap test in the past three years or if you're at risk for
  an STD, getting tested and treated before pregnancy will make
  your pregnancy safer.

+ **Look around your home and work environment for any
  potential toxins.** Limit or eliminate your exposure to X-rays,
  solvents, lead, or other chemicals that may be harmful to a
  developing embryo.

+ **Think about the home into which you will bring your baby.**
  Are there issues such as domestic violence, abuse, or addiction present? Honestly addressing these issues now will save
  you and your baby heartache later.

TRYING TO CONCEIVE

Human beings aren't terribly efficient at reproduction. Pregnancy only happens about 20 percent of the time when sperm is present at the time of ovulation. (You wouldn't think it was that low based on the number of unplanned pregnancies, would you?) Many couples need to try for a few months before pregnancy happens. Ninety percent of healthy couples will conceive within one year of trying if there are no infertility issues present.

If you've been tracking your menstrual cycles, you probably have a good idea when you're ovulating. As mentioned previously there are several smartphone apps have a good reputation for tracking ovulation:

+ CycleBeads: available for Android and Apple devices (www .cyclebeads.com)
+ Fertility Friend: available for Apple devices (www.fertility friend.com)
+ Period Tracker Lite: available for Android and Apple devices
+ iPeriod: available for Android and Apple devices (www.wink pass.com/iperiod.html)

To be even more sure, you can use an ovulation predictor kit available at most drugstores. Testing your urine once each day during days nine to fourteen of your cycle will tell you the twenty-four-hour window during which a mature egg is releasing from your ovary.

If your periods are regular, having intercourse about every other day from days nine to fifteen of your cycle will maximize your chances for getting pregnant. The rest of the month, enjoy intimacy without the pressure of performance. If you're not pregnant within six to twelve months of trying, see your doctor. (We'll discuss infertility in greater detail in chapter 7.)

NUTRITION WHILE PREGNANT

When you're pregnant or trying to conceive, you're eating for two. That doesn't mean you need twice the calories! Even so, everything you place in your body is going to impact not only you, but also the new life growing within you. The nutritional quality of everything you eat becomes important. Make sure the majority of what you eat is nutrient dense—full of protein, vitamins, and minerals. You'll need to significantly limit processed food and junk food if you want your baby to get the very best.

First, drink water. Lots of it. Soft drinks contain too much sugar or artificial sweetener and aren't a good choice during pregnancy. Try flavored water if you need to, but just do it. Water is needed for many things during pregnancy: the extra blood your body is making, the growth of the uterus, the amniotic fluid around the baby, and more. Adequate fluid intake will lessen your risk for dizziness, constipation, urinary tract infections, and premature uterine contractions.

Now for some specific nutrient "problems" during pregnancy.

Iron

During pregnancy, your body makes a lot more blood, which requires iron. Most prenatal vitamins contain some iron, but many women need extra iron during pregnancy to lessen the degree of anemia that often develops. Dark green vegetables, enriched whole-grain bread or cereal, or occasional red meat are good sources of iron.

Calcium

Baby's bones will need a lot of calcium, and baby will take it from *your* bones if you aren't getting enough. Three or four servings daily of calcium-rich foods, such as dairy products, will provide what you need. If you can't or choose not to eat milk products, take 1,000 mg of extra calcium daily.

Eating for Two

When pregnant, keep the following dietary guidelines in mind:

- *Drink plenty of water.*
- *Limit processed food.*
- *Include lean protein with each meal.*
- *Eat plenty of fruits and vegetables.*
- *Choose whole-grain foods.*
- *Include a variety of dairy products.*
- *Don't eat undercooked meat, raw fish, or soft cheese.*
- *Twice-weekly low-mercury fish is OK.*

Protein

Your growing uterus, the placenta, baby, and your extra blood supply all need a lot of protein. Try to make sure you have protein at each meal through dairy products, fish, chicken, eggs, nuts, or legumes such as beans or peas. Low-fat red meat a couple times a week is OK if you choose. Cheese is not a good source of protein by itself because of the high fat content of most cheeses.

Fiber

Your gastrointestinal system thrives on fiber, and you need it even more during pregnancy to limit the constipation many women experience. Fruits, vegetables, whole grains, and legumes are good sources. Make sure you get some at each meal.

Vitamins and minerals

There's no better source for most vitamins and minerals than a wide variety of fruits and vegetables. Choose a variety of colors: red, yellow, dark green, purple. Even so, pregnancy is one time a daily multivitamin makes a lot of sense. And it's a good time to consider Juice Plus+ if you haven't previously. (If you choose Juice Plus+, your doctor may recommend additional folic acid and iron also. See chapter 17 for more information.)

Mercury versus DHA

Fish present a catch-22 for pregnant women. Larger fish, such as shark, swordfish, king mackerel, or tilefish, contain high amounts of mercury, which is detrimental to baby's developing nervous system. However, many fish contain large amounts of omega-3 fatty acids such as DHA (docosahexaenoic acid), which is vital to baby's eye and nervous system development. The best consensus: If you choose to eat fish, choose low-mercury varieties, such as salmon or tilapia, and limit your consumption to two servings a week. It's also smart to choose a prenatal vitamin that includes DHA.

Foodborne infections

Soft cheeses, such as Brie, feta, or Mexican-style cheese, are often unpasteurized and may contain listeria, a bacteria especially detrimental to pregnant women. Hard cheese, cottage cheese, or cream cheese is OK. Undercooked meat can be especially risky during pregnancy. Ideally choose fruits and vegetables that can be washed, peeled, or cooked. Be cautious about the source of any uncooked greens, such as salads.

Sweeteners

Moderate amounts of sugar are probably safest. Saccharin is a no-no during pregnancy, as it can cross the placenta and accumulate in baby's tissues. There is controversy about other artificial sweeteners, such as aspartame and sucralose. If you have a choice, it's probably better to stay away from anything artificial, especially during pregnancy.

Processed foods

Fast food, frozen dinners, baked desserts, and junk snack food may seem appealing during pregnancy, especially when you're hungry but don't otherwise feel great. But pregnancy is not the time to risk eating lower-quality food. Almost every bite you take should be loaded with something valuable, such as protein, calcium, vitamins, or fiber. It's too hard to get enough of those necessary ingredients. That doesn't mean you can't indulge a craving now and then. Plan ahead, have healthy snacks around, and make sure at least 90 percent of your food is healthy.

These nutritional principles are also helpful for women trying to conceive. Before and during pregnancy, make your meals full of colorful fruits and vegetables, lean protein, and whole grains. Your body and your baby will be glad.

EXERCISE DURING PREGNANCY

Being physically active is very helpful during pregnancy. Women who get regular exercise, such as walking, don't gain excessive weight or develop gestational diabetes as often. They also seem to have an easier time during labor and delivery, and some believe labor is quicker in women who have been more physically active.

Most women can safely exercise during pregnancy. If you have bleeding, are at risk for preterm labor, or have certain other complications, your doctor may limit your activity. Two things to be cautious of: 1) your joints become looser because of the hormones of pregnancy, so high-impact exercise such as running will lead to an increased chance of injury; and 2) your baby generates heat your body needs to get rid of, so exercising in a hot environment may be more dangerous for both you and your baby.

Drink plenty of fluids before and after you exercise; it will help maintain blood flow to the placenta and help your body get rid of the extra heat. Don't exercise outdoors in hot weather while pregnant. Limit your exercise to thirty-minute periods of time; that will give you and your baby a chance to recover more effectively.

PRENATAL CARE

There are many sources of information on prenatal care, and this chapter can't address everything you might expect during your pregnancy. But these ideas will help you make appropriate choices during this important time.

You need a health professional to monitor you during pregnancy, whether it's through a prenatal clinic, a nurse midwife, a family practitioner, or an obstetrician. Whom you see is less important than that an experienced professional is watching for preventable problems and catching any problems early. I've seen too many women who didn't get adequate prenatal care end up with problems that might have been prevented or treated before they caused serious complications.

It's important for you and your doctor to know exactly how far along you are in your pregnancy. That is best determined soon after you conceive. When you first know or suspect you may be pregnant, get a medical evaluation right away. An ultrasound during the first trimester (three months) is the most accurate in determining your due date.

Your blood pressure and your baby's growth should be monitored regularly during your pregnancy, more often as your due date gets closer. Whether you need further ultrasounds will be determined between you and your doctor. You'll also need to be tested for gestational diabetes (GDM); if you have GDM, controlling your blood sugar during pregnancy will make the chance of complications much less.

Prenatal diagnosis has become quite popular in the last several years. Until recently, the only way to determine the baby's genetic makeup was to do an amniocentesis—removing fluid from the sac around the baby, usually around sixteen weeks of pregnancy. Then chorionic villus sampling—a biopsy of the developing placenta—became available, which is done around ten to twelve weeks. Today we know that a small amount of baby's DNA is present in mother's blood, which allows doctors to obtain information about baby's genetic makeup from testing a sample of mother's blood. Such blood tests can be done anytime after ten weeks of pregnancy.

Each of these prenatal DNA tests has limitations. None can guarantee 100 percent accuracy, though most give useful information in more than 99 percent of cases. There are usually significant costs involved as well. There is a lot of debate among pregnancy specialists about which women should be encouraged to have prenatal diagnosis and which test is most appropriate in any given circumstance.

If you're over age thirty-five or if you have risk factors in your pregnancy, your doctor will probably bring up the option of prenatal diagnosis. These tests can detect such conditions as Down syndrome, other chromosome problems, and certain other genetic disorders. It's completely your choice whether to have one of these tests or not, and you should ask questions until you understand exactly what the test will look for.

Think also about how you might respond if something abnormal were discovered in your baby's genetic makeup. Some couples feel they wouldn't do anything different, such as terminate the pregnancy, under any circumstance and therefore choose not to undergo such testing. However, if you do choose to have a prenatal diagnosis test, knowing about a problem in advance may help you, your family, and your doctors better prepare for what may happen later in your pregnancy and at delivery. It's a decision only you and your husband can make.

LABOR AND DELIVERY

The moment has come. You're in labor. It won't be long until you'll welcome your brand-new baby. Hopefully you've thought about the decisions you need to make long before the contractions begin.

I've seen too many unexpected problems happen suddenly during labor and delivery, and I can't recommend that you plan to deliver at home or at a separate birthing center. The daughter of a friend of mine had a healthy pregnancy supervised by a compassionate midwife and planned to deliver at home. Unfortunately a problem developed during labor, and by the time the midwife was able to bring her to the hospital, the baby had died. That's only one story, and I could tell others. When an emergency happens, there may be only minutes in which to act to save the baby's life, and sometimes the mother's as well.

It has become fashionable for soon-to-be moms to create a birth plan, a document outlining what they want and don't want during labor and delivery. Thinking through how you want to be cared for during this time is a great idea, but I encourage you to consider your birth plan a work in progress. The outcome you want—a healthy baby—may sometimes necessitate measures you had hoped to avoid. Make your plan, but don't get too stressed if some deviation from your plan becomes necessary. If your doctor recommends something you don't want, pause and ask questions. Make sure you understand the reason behind his or her suggestion, and then work together to get to a safe delivery for you and your baby.

Troublesome Pregnancy Symptoms

You may feel great during much of your pregnancy. Pregnant women really do have a wonderful "glow" about them. But you may also struggle with some unpleasant symptoms. Here are some ways to deal with some of them.

Morning sickness

Some nausea and occasional vomiting is present in most pregnancies and usually subsides after the first trimester, or around fourteen to sixteen weeks. Dry food such as crackers, seltzer water or ginger ale, and frequent small meals may be sufficient to curb the symptoms. Supplements of vitamin B6, ginger, or peppermint may help. A newly approved prescription medication, Diclegis, is very helpful for women whose symptoms can't be controlled otherwise. If you have severe hyperemesis gravidarum, you may need to be admitted to the hospital for IV fluids and, occasionally, IV nutrition. There is a silver lining to all this nausea, though: morning sickness is usually a reassuring sign of a healthy pregnancy.

Constipation

Pregnancy hormones decrease the motility of your gastrointestinal tract, and your growing uterus places more pressure on your colon. Iron often prescribed during pregnancy is also constipating. Lots of fluids, exercise, and fiber in fruits, vegetables, and whole grains will help. If necessary, it's OK to take occasional laxatives or stool softeners.

General aches and pains

Your joints are looser, your center of gravity is changing, and you're carrying around more weight. All that can lead to aches and pains in your back, pelvis, joints, and elsewhere. Gentle exercise, including stretching, a heating pad on your back, or resting with extra pillows may help. Consider a maternity support belt to relieve some of the weight pulling on your back and pelvis. And if you ever think you might be having contractions, contact your doctor right away.

Emotional stress

During pregnancy, your brain is flooded with hormones it's not used to processing. Your body feels different. It is normal to have emotional swings and feel less able to handle stress than you did when you weren't pregnant. Get extra rest, plenty of exercise, and good quality food. Ask your husband or a good friend for support if you need it. Give yourself some grace, and please ask for help if you feel unable to handle any anxious feelings or depression during your pregnancy.

This has been a necessarily brief overview of your health related to pregnancy. I hope your planning for parenthood and your experience of pregnancy is one of the best times of your life.

When I deliver a baby, I often tell the excited parents, "Every new life is a miracle from God." Treasure that miracle.

Congratulations, Mommy!

A FEW QUESTIONS

Q: Can a vegetarian have a healthy pregnancy?

A: Absolutely. You'll need to pay extra attention to getting adequate protein, but nuts, legumes, and dairy products can do the job just fine. If you don't use dairy products, you'll need extra calcium (see above). And if you're a true vegan, you may need to consider extra protein supplements also.

Q: I'm scared about getting pregnant, and about delivery. Can I do anything to help myself feel less worried?

A: As one young soon-to-be mom said, "Growing a human is hard work!" Know that for thousands of years mothers have felt anxious about everything related to having a baby. Usually everything turns out great. Do all you can to be healthy before you get pregnant, and take care of yourself while carrying your baby. Most of all, remember that a new baby is God's opinion that the world should go on. He's got you, and your baby, in His hands.

Chapter 7

ALL ABOUT INFERTILITY

S OMETHING DEEP WITHIN a woman's soul makes her want to be a mother. Sure, there's the biological need to pass on your genetic heritage and continue the human race. But it's more than that. A woman feels validated in her femininity when she becomes pregnant, feels her child grow and move within her, and brings that child into the world at the time of birth—and that's only the beginning of what being a mother means.

Let me say right here that if you've chosen not to be a mother, that's OK. There's nothing wrong with you. But for the up to 15 percent of women who aren't able to have a child when they wish, infertility often becomes the defining characteristic of how they see themselves. If that's you, you know how easily the pursuit of pregnancy can take over your thoughts, your marriage, your schedule, your finances—indeed, your whole life.

TEST for Pregnancy

Four factors that must come together for a normal pregnancy to occur:

- *Tubes*
- *Eggs*
- *Sperm*
- *Timing*

Helping infertile couples build their families has been one of the primary joys and biggest challenges of my medical career. I've rejoiced at the moment of a positive pregnancy test for some. I've seen the delight in parents' eyes when they return to share their newborn bundle of joy with me. And I've shared tears of disappointment with others.

We know so much more about the biology of reproduction than ever before. There are exciting medical advances in infertility treatments that may help, and there are some steps you can take on your own. There are some heavy ethical challenges involved as well.

GETTING PREGNANT

Four basic components (using the acronym TEST) must function properly for a normal pregnancy to happen.

Tubes (and other anatomy). All the anatomical elements of a woman's reproductive system are important for pregnancy. The fallopian tubes must be open, free of scar tissue, and able to move freely in order to bring the egg and sperm together. Contractions in the wall of the uterus and fallopian tubes are important in helping the egg and sperm find each other. And the uterus must provide a mature, healthy environment for an early embryo to attach, establish its blood supply with mom, and grow.

Eggs. A baby girl is born with all the egg cells she will ever have. (This has recently been challenged scientifically, but in general it's true.) Reproductive hormones must induce a healthy, mature egg cell to be released from the ovary at just the right time. That egg cell must have the proper genetic code to develop into a healthy human being. And the egg must contain the proper elements needed to nourish an early embryo during the first several days after conception until a connection with mom's blood supply can be established.

Sperm. Many couples don't realize how often a "male factor" is involved in infertility. Sperm have a difficult task. The winning sperm cell must win the race against potentially millions of others, making its way through the cervical mucus, uterine cavity, and fallopian tubes to find the single egg cell—and it must do so within a few hours after the egg is released. It must attach to and penetrate the thick wall of the egg, which then changes instantly to prevent any other sperm from entering.

Timing. Healthy sperm must meet mature egg within a window of time lasting only a few hours. Sometimes because of busy or conflicting schedules, difficulty with intercourse, or other reasons, couples may struggle to have intercourse regularly during the time of ovulation.

There are also a number of less visible factors necessary for a pregnancy to occur. There are hundreds, probably thousands, of genes that only function during conception and early pregnancy. And a woman's immune system, which normally fights foreign invaders such

Dr. Carol Says . . .

"Every new life is a miracle from God."

as harmful bacteria and viruses, must recognize that this embryo is desired and switch from fighting it to protecting it.

When you realize how many factors go into establishing a healthy pregnancy, you can see how the birth of a child is a miracle every time. I hope I never cease to be amazed. Every new life truly is a miracle from God.

"WHY AM I INFERTILE?"

Human beings aren't terribly efficient at reproduction. Even if everything is perfect, pregnancy doesn't happen every time a couple has intercourse. The chance of a young, healthy couple conceiving during any given month is only about 20 percent. Up to 90 percent of such couples will conceive during one year of trying.

Health Tip

If you're overweight, losing 10 to 15 percent of your body weight will improve ovulation and make pregnancy easier and healthier.

Infertility is defined as the failure to conceive after one year of attempting pregnancy and not using any contraception. There are several general categories of infertility. In roughly one-third of couples, there is a problem with ovulation. The chance that poor egg quality is affecting fertility becomes increasingly common as a woman moves closer to age forty and beyond. In another roughly 25 percent, there may be some anatomical problem, such as endometriosis, damage to the fallopian tubes, or an abnormal uterine cavity. In up to 40 percent of couples, there is inadequate function or quantity of sperm—a male factor. In 25 percent or more of couples, more than one infertility factor may be involved. For 10 to 20 percent of couples, no specific cause can be found, so-called unexplained infertility. (For more facts on infertility, check out ReproductiveFacts.org.)

Remember TEST—tubes, eggs, sperm, and timing. Here are some of the more common symptoms that indicate a possible reason for infertility in each category:

+ Tubes and other anatomy: a history of sexually transmitted infection; significant pain with periods or intercourse; previous abdominal or pelvic surgery

+ Eggs: problems with ovulation, including irregular or absent menstrual periods; obesity; being over age thirty-five; smoking
+ Sperm: difficulty with sexual performance; tobacco, alcohol, or drug use
+ Timing: inability to have regular intercourse during the time of ovulation

That still leaves many couples who have no idea why pregnancy isn't happening for them—and that's when infertility testing can provide some answers.

"What Can I Do to Help This?"

While every new life is a miracle, there are some things you can do to help that miracle come into being. Some involve your general health and lifestyle, and others specifically involve trying to get pregnant. The following lifestyle choices clearly affect fertility.

Control your weight.

Some women's reproductive systems are very sensitive to changes in body weight. I have seen so many patients who are overweight and have associated problems with ovulation, and I tell all of them the same thing: If you lose just 10 to 15 percent of your body weight, it may significantly improve your ovulation rate. This means, for instance, if you weigh three hundred pounds, the goal would be to lose thirty pounds.

Some women conceive on their own simply by losing weight. Losing weight will also increase the success of any fertility treatment you may choose and make your future pregnancy easier and healthier. The closer you can get to your ideal weight, the better. But remember, even small amounts of weight loss really do make a difference.

Quit smoking and other harmful substances.

Tobacco is especially toxic to eggs, so much so that 13 percent of

> **Health Tip**
>
> *Moderate coffee or tea use (one to two cups per day) is OK while trying to get pregnant. Heavy use (three to five cups per day) may decrease your fertility rate and affect the health of your pregnancy later.*

infertility can be attributed to smoking. Smokers go through meno-pause earlier, meaning their eggs are older than their biological age. Smoking affects the success rate of infertility treatment so much that some infertility centers require a woman to stop smoking prior to undergoing more advanced fertility treatments, such as IVF. Smoking is also toxic to sperm, but alcohol and other drugs are even more so. I remember a patient whose husband completely reversed his low sperm count by quitting alcohol and marijuana and losing some extra weight. By the way, moderate coffee or tea use is probably OK.

Optimize management of other illnesses.

Women with diabetes, thyroid problems, or a seizure disorder face special challenges getting pregnant. If you have one of these illnesses or any medical problem requiring you to be on regular medication, see a fertility specialist before trying to conceive. Being on too little or too much thyroid hormone replacement may decrease your fertility. Some anti-seizure medications are especially toxic to embryos, and you may need to switch medications. And diabetes must be tightly controlled prior to conceiving to minimize the chance for serious birth defects.

Take vitamins.

What's in your body at the time you conceive makes a big differ-ence in the health of your baby. Many organ systems in the devel-oping embryo have already begun to form by the time you have a positive pregnancy test. Begin taking prenatal vitamins as soon as you start trying to conceive. Instead of a commercial vitamin, you might choose a phytonutrient supplement, such as Juice Plus+. (See chapter 17 for more on this subject.)

Consider supplements.

The only supplement I can recommend for infertility is myoino-sitol. A variety of recent studies show that women taking myoinositol and folic acid ovulate more regularly, have a shorter time to concep-tion, and possibly respond better to fertility treatments. You can find generic myoinositol or purchase the branded Pregnitude; aim for 2 grams (2,000 mg) twice daily. This supplement is most useful for women in whom an ovulation disorder is the cause for their decreased fertility.

Take care of your body.

If there's ever a time to take care of yourself, it's while you are trying to conceive. Eating a healthy diet of plenty of fruits, vegetables, and healthy protein, limiting processed and junk food, getting appropriate exercise, and managing your stress well are always good health habits. If you're having a difficult time conceiving, these general health measures may just give your body the boost you need to get pregnant.

Acknowledge your biological clock.

Fertility becomes increasingly difficult as a woman gets closer to forty and beyond. More women are delaying childbearing for personal reasons, including career, and there's nothing wrong with that. That doesn't mean you should have a child at twenty-five if you're not ready, but don't expect your fertility to be the same in ten or fifteen years. Pregnancy in a woman's later thirties and forties also carries increased risks of chromosomal problems and pregnancy complications.

The biological clock is real. A woman's best chance of getting pregnant is during her early twenties, when her reproductive system is mature and her eggs are fresh. Her fertility begins to decline significantly during her midthirties. By age forty, her chance of getting pregnant is only 20 percent or less of what it was in her twenties, and each year after that, her fertility dramatically declines even further.

> ### Dr. Carol Says...
>
> *"I believe up to half of infertile couples might be able to get pregnant simply by following healthy lifestyle measures consistently."*

Even though some women do conceive in their forties, "old eggs" are a tough challenge to overcome.

These measures may not seem like much, but they do make a difference. I don't have one specific study to prove it, but I believe up to half of infertile couples might be able to get pregnant simply by conscientiously following these lifestyle measures over a period of time.

TRYING TO CONCEIVE

Pregnancy can't happen without sperm and egg getting together at the right time. How do you know when you're ovulating? And how often should you have intercourse?

Counting cycle days becomes important when you're trying to conceive. Doctors consider the first day of your menstrual cycle to be Day 1. Don't count spotting that sometimes begins before your period; the first day of menstrual flow is Day 1.

For a woman who has menstrual cycles every twenty-eight days, ovulation usually occurs around Day 14. An ovulation predictor kit can help confirm when a mature egg is releasing. Many brands are available without a prescription at most drugstores. Some women enjoy the digital kits that help you track your cycle days and show a smiley face on your most fertile days, but less expensive kits will be just as helpful in telling you when you're ovulating.

Look for an ovulation predictor kit that is designed to detect the LH surge. Approximately thirty-six hours prior to ovulation, the pituitary gland begins to pump out large amounts of luteinizing hormone (LH). That signals the ovary to release the mature egg—the moment of ovulation. If the egg isn't fertilized within twelve to twenty-four hours, it deteriorates and the ovary prepares for next month. Testing your urine once each day with an ovulation predictor kit is usually more than 95 percent accurate in detecting the day of ovulation.

Cycle Schedule for Attempting Pregnancy

- *Note and record Day 1.*
- *Begin ovulation kit testing on Day 10.*
- *Have intercourse every other day from Day 10 until ovulation.*
- *Take a pregnancy test fourteen days after ovulation.*

Although healthy sperm may survive in a woman's reproductive tract for several days, having more and fresher sperm present gives Mr. Right a better chance of meeting Mrs. Egg and establishing a healthy pregnancy. Having intercourse every day or every other day around ovulation provides the maximum chance of pregnancy. Having intercourse more often than this will not improve your chances further.

When your ovulation kit turns positive, make sure sperm is there. If you haven't had intercourse in the previous twenty-four hours, plan to do so that day. Then relax. Record the day, and plan to do a pregnancy test in fourteen days. And while you're waiting, enjoy intimacy without having to perform in trying to get pregnant. Enjoy some time focusing on your relationship with your husband.

Note: Basal body temperature charting has been extensively used in the past but is time-consuming, less accurate, and less reliable in predicting ovulation. It is not generally recommended for couples attempting pregnancy today.

INFERTILITY TESTING AND TREATMENT

There are three times you should see a doctor for help with infertility:

+ You've been trying for one year or more without success.
+ You know or suspect you have a medical problem affecting your fertility, such as irregular or absent menstrual periods.
+ You're over age thirty-five. In that case, seek care if you've been trying for six months without success.

Some ob-gyns have a special interest in infertility and are able to provide basic infertility testing. I also encourage you to see a reproductive endocrinologist sooner rather than later, as they have completed subspecialty training and certification that includes infertility testing and treatment. Your regular ob-gyn may suggest a referral, or you can search for a specialist at the American Society for Reproductive Medicine's website at www.asrm.org/findamember.

When you see a fertility specialist, expect the initial tests evaluating eggs, sperm, and anatomy to be completed within one month. Those initial tests should give you and your doctor the information necessary to plan an initial course of treatment.

There are three basic levels of infertility treatment: oral medications, injectable medications, and assisted reproductive technologies (ART) such as in vitro fertilization (IVF). Each level involves increasing expense, increasing risk, and increasing time commitment. But each level also provides an increased chance for successfully conceiving. Appendix A outlines the typical tests used in an infertility workup and describes the three levels of infertility treatment in more detail. You can progress as slow or as fast through the process as you wish. And most important, you can stop at any time.

Third-Party Reproduction
and Genetic Issues

The subject of third-party reproduction—that of using a third party to bring about a baby—always generates considerable controversy. For a single woman or a woman whose husband has poor or absent sperm, donor sperm can be inseminated directly into her uterus or used for IVF. A woman whose eggs are too old or unhealthy can undergo IVF using donor eggs from a young, healthy woman. In both of these instances, the "intended mother" is able to experience pregnancy and delivery.

In yet another option, a surrogate mother carries the child for the "intended parents." She can become pregnant through insemination using the intended father's sperm and thereby provide both the egg and the uterus. Or she can become pregnant through a transfer of embryos formed by eggs and sperm from the intended parents, thus providing only the uterus. As you might imagine, this option brings with it the most intense legal and ethical issues.

In vitro fertilization and third-party reproduction are sometimes used when the mother or father has a genetic condition that they don't wish to pass on to their children. Using donor eggs or donor sperm bypasses the genetic problem completely. With IVF, a couple's early embryos can be tested for a range of genetic problems, with only normal embryos transferred. The possible genetic conditions that can be tested and the various technologies available to do so are expanding rapidly. This is one of the most exciting areas in medical science today.

However, just because something is medically possible doesn't always mean it's wise to do, ethical, or consistent with your faith. I provide some comments below that may help you think through some of these challenging issues.

Psychological Impact

Couples facing infertility are on a painful and frustrating journey. Some women face regret at waiting so long to have a family or feel guilt over a past abortion or sexually transmitted infection that affects fertility now. Some men feel a serious threat to their manhood when a male factor is discovered in the process. Both men and women may feel like their body has become an enemy rather than a friend.

Infertility can also present significant stress to a marriage. Sex becomes a matter of performance, and having "sex on demand" to achieve a pregnancy can become

Dr. Carol Says...

"You're in charge! Don't get on the infertility roller coaster."

difficult for both partners. The ability to enjoy intimacy and truly feel connected can seem impossible, even when having sex for "fun" and not for getting pregnant.

Many women feel like infertility becomes a roller coaster they can't exit. You're counting cycle days and maintaining your calendar. Your hopes rise each month, only to fall flat when your next period begins. You go for infertility testing and treatment, and there's always one more thing to try. One more month of medication. One more insemination. Somehow you'll find the money for one more cycle of IVF. One more side effect. One more blood test. One more injection. Your body becomes a thing to be managed. Maybe *this* will be the time you finally get pregnant, you think.

Here are a few important things to remember as you cope with infertility and any treatment you choose:

1. **You are more than your ability to get pregnant.** Your desire to conceive and deliver a child is God-given. It's part of what makes you a woman. But you're also much more than that. You're a wife, a friend, perhaps a sister, a coworker, an artist, a businesswoman, or some other beautiful, important human being. And most of all, you're a child of God. Focusing on and nurturing the other parts of yourself is critically important, even as you continue to hope and pray for a child.

2. **You are in charge.** Don't get on the roller coaster! You get to decide how long to try, when to take a break, how much time and money to invest, and how far to go with treatment—if at all. You get to choose what treatments are right for you and your family and are consistent with your faith. It's OK to stop. It's OK

to start again if you wish. It's OK to say no to something you don't want or to change your mind.

3. **Take care of your marriage.** Infertility and its treatment often bring a great deal of stress to a marriage.
   It's important to take care of your relationship and
   each other. I've seen some marriages deteriorate under
   the burden of infertility and fall apart just when pregnancy finally happens. Do what it takes to keep your
   marriage strong. You want your home to be ready to
   welcome a child if God so blesses you. And take time
   to enjoy intimacy, including sex completely separate
   from trying to conceive.

4. **Get support.** If your husband fully supports you, be
   grateful. It's also helpful to get together with other
   women struggling with infertility. Resolve is a national
   organization advocating for infertility and its treatment. They have chapters in many local communities and provide resources, information, and support
   at www.resolve.org. Seeing a therapist or counselor
   who understands infertility may help you manage the
   stress and decision making involved in infertility too.
   It's OK to ask for and get some help.

ETHICAL ISSUES

Some infertility treatments present significant concerns for people of
faith. Are we playing God by using infertility treatment? Is fertilizing
eggs and sperm in the laboratory using IVF against God's plan? Is
third-party reproduction ever OK? Is it OK for a woman without a
husband to get pregnant?

As a Christian and as a minister, I've wrestled with some of these
issues personally, and I know how difficult they can be to work
through. As a result of my own faith journey and relationship with
God, there are things some other physicians do that I've chosen not
to do. My purpose here is not to give theological pronouncements but
to provide a framework and perspective for you to think about and
pray through the questions on your own.

Fertility is one of our natural biological functions as human beings.

Becoming pregnant and bringing a child into the world is a God-given desire most women have. Children are a blessing from God. (See Psalm 127:4–5.)

But pregnancy is not a right. A child is not a thing you can buy. There's no law, human or divine, guaranteeing every person should, or can, have a child just because they want one. Like the need and desire for food or pleasure, the need and desire for a baby is healthy, but it can become unbalanced or distorted. And it can be met in either healthy or unhealthy ways.

In Scripture God looked kindly on women struggling with infertility and sometimes blessed them with a child. (See Genesis 21:1–2, 1 Samuel 1, and Luke 1:7–13.) I believe God looks kindly on couples striving to bring a child into the world today. Using infertility treatments—including IVF, if a couple so desires—can be consistent with God's design.

Some, especially the Catholic Church, have argued that IVF separates the unitive and procreative aspects of intercourse and is thus against God's plan. As in the discussion of contraception in chapter 5, I believe there is another biblical view. Using IVF to have a child does not negate a married couple's unity or their joint actions in procreation. The location where an embryo is formed (i.e., in the laboratory) is not a moral issue. If a couple has peace with God in jointly pursuing IVF and has a clear plan for any extra embryos (see below), God can bless IVF as a means to build their family.

The biblical values to consider in this discussion include the importance of both mother and father in a child's life and both parents' commitment to provide for and raise that child. Although the desire for a child is God-given, prospective parents must consider whether they have the financial, emotional, and family resources to raise a child well. Many children are born into circumstances that don't provide that ideal support, but choosing to create a child when one knows they can't provide what that child needs in all areas is irresponsible and inconsistent with God's design.

Bringing a third party into the equation by using a donor egg, donor sperm, or surrogate may not be sinful. But is it wise? These arrangements risk creating prob-

> **God Values Life!**
>
> Before I formed you in the womb, I knew you.
>
> —JEREMIAH 1:5

lems, such as family conflict and emotional difficulties for both adults and children involved. Prospective parents and society argue about these interventions, and they have become big business. In my opinion it's usually wisest to avoid third-party reproduction because of the unnecessary risk of pain it brings to the children involved. Might there be times when genetic problems in a prospective parent might make donor eggs or sperm a good option? Medically, yes. Spiritually, I would encourage you to wrestle with God deeply in prayer and only proceed if you have solid peace in doing so. Embryo or child adoption are certainly other options.

You may have already guessed my position on some of the most controversial issues of all. I believe God intended children to be raised by a father and a mother in a committed marriage. Some children aren't blessed to have this type of family, but it's still God's plan. Living according to this truth would prevent unmarried women or same-sex couples from undergoing infertility treatment. This may not be a popular position, but it's the only one I believe is supported by Scripture and is in the best interest of the children involved.

IVF treatment often results in more embryos than are necessary to achieve pregnancy. Because God values life—all life—a clear plan must be in place for how to handle any extra embryos. If a couple doesn't desire to use them to try to have another child, one good option is embryo donation.[1] And adopting embryos would also be a graceful way to build a family if a couple wishes to do so.

What you've read in this section is certainly controversial. You'll hear preachers, fertility specialists, and parents' and women's rights groups express other opinions on every side. I encourage you to take time to be thoughtful in making your decisions. Remember that as painful as infertility is to you, having a child must be about the child and not about you. It's a matter for much thoughtful prayer.

Because of the strong desire you may have for a child, it's easy to forget that this isn't really about you. Your infertility journey also impacts your husband and other family members. And it most certainly impacts any child you would bring into the world.

Don't have a child simply for your own benefit, because it's your "right," or because it's something you want. Parenting demands more from you than any other job you'll ever take on. Babies grow up and bring you both joy and heartache. And raising a child is far too much stress to add to a troubled marriage.

Instead have a child because you and your husband want to unselfishly pour out your lives into another human being, because you have so much love to give away that you can't imagine your family being complete any other way. Having a child can be a wonderful journey that can bring you and your husband together if you both desire it. Unity of purpose with your husband and the peace of God are priceless as you work to achieve pregnancy. If that's you, enjoy the journey to express the creative power God built within you to bring a new human being into the world.

A FEW QUESTIONS

Q: Where does adoption fit into infertility treatment, medically and ethically?

A: Adopting an embryo, baby, child, or teen is a wonderful expression of love that mirrors God's love toward us. (See biblical passages such as Romans 8:15 and Ephesians 1:5.) Some may wonder why I view adoption so positively while I express real reservations about third-party reproduction arrangements. With adoption, you as a couple are choosing to extend your heart and home to a child who has already been brought into being by someone else who is now unwilling or unable to provide further parenting. Ethically I believe that is in a very different category from choosing to create a child through third-party reproduction.

There are many possible reasons to choose adoption: not wanting to pass on a genetic illness to a child, failure of infertility treatment to result in a live birth, or making the choice not to invest the time and money into such treatment. Adoptive families do have challenges, but it can be a beautiful way to share your love with those who need it so badly.

Q: Does infertility treatment affect a mother's health in the future?

A: Some older, controversial studies concluded that repeated treatment with ovulation-inducing medications may increase a woman's chances for developing ovarian cancer. More recent reviews have called that conclusion into question. Some causes of infertility itself may somewhat increase a woman's chances for ovarian cancer, which makes this question even more difficult. One large, recent review concluded that there is no convincing evidence of such a connection, though more study is needed. Ovulation induction medications may slightly increase the risk of borderline ovarian tumors, which do not act the same as malignant ovarian cancer.[2]

Chapter 8
WHEN MENOPAUSE BEGINS

YOU ARE LIKELY to live one-third of your life after menopause. Just think of all the things you *won't* have to worry about during that time!

I'm glad to be a member of the over-fifty club. I seriously don't think fifty is old. And I don't know if I'll feel any older at sixty. I know women in their seventies who are living fuller and more active lives than most of the rest of us. There is a lot of truth to the adage "You're only as old as you feel."

As freeing and productive as the senior years can be, the hormone changes women experience can bring some complications. Menopause has also become big business—just look at the success of whole pharmacies full of products promoted to help women with the symptoms of menopause. Sadly evidence behind many of these products is gravely lacking, and women spend a lot of money for things that aren't helpful or are perhaps even harmful.

If you haven't already, pause to celebrate and enjoy the thought of no more periods, no more birth control, no more menstrual calendars, no more pads or tampons, no more pregnancy worries, and no more PMS. You're free!

Now, let's get down to business and deal with the troublesome symptoms that may appear during and after menopause.

STARTING THE CHANGE

The word *menopause* means "a woman's final menstrual period." There is no way to know if any given period is your final one until long after the fact. Most women have changes in their menstrual pattern prior to menopause, and time is the only way to know for sure if you're there. No periods for one year, along with the decline in ovarian hormones, means you've reached menopause.

But as any woman knows who has gone through menopause, the symptoms don't begin or end on any single day. The climacteric transition is the period of time during which ovarian function declines and then stops. For most women, it lasts for a few years, and some symptoms may begin well before a woman's final period.

There is a wide variation in the age of menopause and what symptoms women experience. If you know about when your mother experienced menopause and what symptoms she had, you'll have some idea of what to expect for yourself, though that can still vary. A woman's periods usually become progressively less regular during her forties. Some become heavier and closer together, while other women simply have lighter periods that come less and less frequently until they finally stop. A woman's final period comes, on average, at age fifty-one.

The above description is true for women going through "natural menopause." But if your ovaries are removed surgically or you undergo a treatment that damages your ovaries, such as chemotherapy, you may go through menopause earlier. The more sudden and complete drop in ovarian hormones often leads to more significant menopausal symptoms immediately.

The most notable change in hormones at menopause is the drop in estrogen. Once a woman's eggs are gone, her ovaries only produce about 10 percent of the estrogen they did previously. That drop in estrogen produces most of the symptoms of menopause. Women may also experience many other symptoms at this time of life that aren't related to the drop in estrogen. It can be helpful to distinguish between what is and what isn't related to the loss of estrogen.

Symptom	Related to loss of estrogen?
Hot flashes	Yes
Night sweats	Probably
Trouble sleeping	Probably
Vaginal dryness	Yes
Discomfort with intercourse	Yes
Thinning hair	Probably not
Tiredness, lack of energy	Only indirectly
Weight gain	No
Loss of muscle tone, especially in pelvic area	Possibly, only in part
Loss of bladder control	Probably not

Symptom	Related to loss of estrogen?
Loss of bone mineral	Yes
Extra facial hair	Only indirectly
Skin changes	Partially
Change in sexual desire	Only indirectly
Change in mood	Only indirectly
Change in thinking (cognition)	Only indirectly

The timing of these symptoms might lead you to think they're all related to declining estrogen, but that isn't necessarily so. We know this by looking at studies comparing women who are given hormone treatment containing estrogen with women who are not. Some of these changes happen regardless of what a woman's estrogen levels are and whether or not women are taking estrogen.

We've only hinted at the possible mental and emotional symptoms related to menopause. That's a topic in itself, and a whole section in chapter 20 is devoted to the "menopause brain."

Many women go through menopause with little or no distress. If that's you, be glad. If you are troubled with menopausal symptoms, though, let's talk about some of the treatment options available.

HORMONE THERAPY

This is the big one, and it has created plenty of controversy. I have one friend, now in her seventies, who has said, "They'll have to pry my Premarin from my cold, dead hands!" I know other women who flatly refuse to consider any hormone treatment, regardless of their symptoms. I think the best solution lies somewhere in the middle.

Estrogen is not a fountain of youth. That is why it's important to consider what changes are related to a decrease in estrogen and which aren't, as in the chart above. There is no treatment available either by prescription, over the counter, or in a supplement that is as effective in decreasing hot flashes and maintaining the elasticity and moisture of the vagina as estrogen is. That doesn't mean other treatments may not be helpful, but nothing will duplicate what estrogen does for those two problems.

Will estrogen help other symptoms? Possibly. You may sleep better. You may notice your skin feels and looks healthier. Some women feel better about sex while taking estrogen, perhaps because intercourse is no longer uncomfortable or because they're sleeping better and feel less fatigued. Some women feel they can think more clearly and are less moody when taking estrogen. These other improvements are harder to predict because so many other things besides estrogen may affect these symptoms. Whatever is related to a drop in estrogen at menopause in your particular case may well improve with hormone therapy.

Hormone therapy does not cause weight gain. Women often gain weight during the menopause transition, but that weight gain is the same whether or not they take hormones. Your metabolism is going through big changes during your forties and fifties, and this is the most likely reason so many women gain weight. You may have to make other lifestyle changes in order to keep your weight under control, even if you didn't have to do so in years past.

As with any medication, estrogen therapy carries some risks. Many women are concerned about breast cancer. There are dozens of studies, some of them very large, looking at this question, and many of them come to different conclusions. My summary of the scientific evidence is this: if estrogen does increase the risk of breast cancer, it's a small increase, and it's probably related primarily to synthetic estrogens taken for five years or more. You should obtain regular mammograms while taking hormone therapy. This doesn't mean you will or won't get breast cancer; it only means estrogen therapy will be a very minor component of that risk.

If you still have your uterus, any estrogen will increase the risk of endometrial cancer (cancer of the lining of the uterus). Unless you've had a hysterectomy, you should also take some progestin (such as progesterone) to decrease that risk.

Other risks are less common. The amount of estrogen prescribed for menopausal symptoms is perhaps 20 percent or less of the amount of estrogen in birth control pills. However, small risks of blood clots, gallstones, or other problems do exist.

What about cardiovascular disease? The Women's Health Initiative (WHI) was a large, well-publicized study that began in 1991 and which, among other things, evaluated the health risks related to postmenopausal hormone therapy.[1] The primary portion of this study was halted in 2002 because of a small increase in breast cancer, heart disease, and stroke among women taking hormone therapy. Many women stopped taking hormone therapy when the initial WHI study results were announced. But it's important to know that the majority of these women started hormone therapy at age sixty or older and weren't using it to treat menopausal symptoms. The risks are not the same for women who use "natural" estrogen and who use it to treat symptoms around the time of menopause (say, age fifty).

By "natural" estrogen, I mean estrogen molecules that are identical to what your ovary made. Other commonly prescribed estrogens, including synthetic estrogens, conjugated estrogens (such as in Premarin), and even plant estrogens are not molecules your body made, is making now, or is used to. These other estrogens may exist in nature, but not in the human body. There is some evidence to support the view that "natural" estrogens provide the least risks. Estradiol is the primary estrogen your ovaries made while they were working, and several commercially available products contain this very molecule.

Not every woman should take estrogen. For those who choose to do so, there are ways to make therapy safer. A lot of data supports the view that "natural" estrogen started around the time of menopause may decrease a woman's risk for cardiovascular disease. This difference likely has to do with the health of a woman's heart and vascular system at the time she begins estrogen therapy. Starting therapy early may protect a woman's heart, while starting later (say, age sixty) is more likely to be harmful. The explanation is likely similar for estrogen's impact on the brain—your risk for dementia, Alzheimer's disease, and the like.

There has been a lot of buzz about bioidentical hormones for treating menopause. The claim is that these hormones are safer than standard prescriptions. The word *bioidentical* is misleading. Many people use it to refer to a compounded hormone product, sometimes combining estradiol, estriol, and estrone—three different estrogen molecules. But what *bioidentical* really means is a hormone identical to what your own body makes or was making. Several FDA-approved prescription products containing estradiol—identical to what your ovaries were making—are available. There is no evidence that adding other estrogen molecules makes this therapy any safer or more effective than using estradiol alone.

I almost exclusively prescribe estradiol to my patients who need hormone therapy for menopausal symptoms. It is available as an oral tablet, skin patch, skin gel, skin spray, vaginal ring, vaginal tablet, or vaginal cream. So take your pick. Some forms also contain a progestin (necessary for women who still have a uterus). There may be some benefit to choosing a non-oral form when possible, as oral estrogen affects production of certain proteins in the liver, while other forms do so much less.

Side effects of estrogen therapy may include breast tenderness or vaginal bleeding. If these develop, your doctor will recommend other tests, such as a mammogram, pelvic ultrasound, or endometrial biopsy (biopsy of the uterine lining). Most women can continue taking hormone therapy after making sure there are no serious problems.

This discussion of hormone therapy has been extensive because it's one of the biggest questions I get asked and because so many women have misconceptions about menopausal hormone therapy. But other measures can also be helpful during menopause.

PROGESTIN THERAPY

If you're not ovulating, you're not making progesterone. And if you're taking any form of estrogen and still have your uterus, you'll need some progestin to block estrogen's action on the continued growth of the uterine lining. Taking progestin for ten to fourteen days each month often leads to repeated light vaginal bleeding similar to periods. Not much fun if you're menopausal! Many women take a smaller dose of progestin daily and may have no vaginal bleeding at all.

Synthetic progestins have been most commonly used and are probably mostly OK. However, some data suggests that the synthetic progestins in medications such as Prempro may be responsible for the small increase in breast cancer risk. In that light, and with a view toward "natural is generally better," progesterone—the same molecule your ovaries used to make—is probably ideal. Prometrium is a commercially available natural progesterone tablet; it's what I prescribe for my postmenopausal patients who need hormone therapy and still have a uterus. Vaginal progesterone is also available as a cream, though it's quite expensive.

Wild yam cream has been promoted as a progesterone treatment, but it's not effective. The human body doesn't have the enzymes needed to convert the precursor molecule in wild yam into progesterone.

ANDROGENS

A woman's ovaries also make androgens (male hormones, principally testosterone), and how much they make decreases at menopause by about 50 percent. If a woman undergoes menopause because her ovaries are surgically removed, this decrease is even greater. Whether or not testosterone is needed during menopause is somewhat controversial.

Those who advocate for testosterone therapy believe it improves women's sense of well-being, energy levels, and sex drive. It also has significant side effects, including weight gain, oily skin, excess hair growth, and sometimes voice changes.

Testosterone is one of many things that can affect a woman's sex drive and sexual response, and a tiny bit goes a long way. For most menopausal women, the risks of testosterone therapy outweigh the possible small benefits. However, if a woman's ovaries have been removed, or in a few other cases, very small amounts of testosterone may be somewhat helpful in making sexual arousal easier.

There's no FDA-approved product providing the small doses of testosterone women would need. Your doctor can prescribe a small percentage of the dose men would take in a gel or cream. You'll need careful monitoring if you choose to try this therapy.

HERBAL/NATURAL PRODUCTS

Late-night television, women's magazines, and the Internet are full of advertisements promoting a variety of "natural" products to menopausal women, promising risk-free and almost immediate relief of menopausal symptoms, weight gain, moodiness, and more. If only it were that easy!

When talking about supplements such as these, it's important to remember the placebo effect: if a person believes something will improve symptoms, it is likely to be beneficial even if there is no active ingredient in the product. Menopausal symptoms respond strongly to the placebo effect. That's why studies of both medications and supplements can be so difficult to interpret well and why any claim that a product is helpful must be supported by research comparing the product with a placebo. A medication or product can only be considered effective if it improves symptoms significantly more than the placebo does.

Many supplements have been touted as helpful for menopausal symptoms, but when compared with a placebo, none of them show consistent benefit. That doesn't always mean you shouldn't try them. Here's a brief summary of the more commonly recommended supplements:

- **Black cohosh.** Possibly decreases hot flashes. There is some concern that it may cause liver problems over time.
- **Flaxseed, flaxseed oil.** Possibly helps with night sweats.
- **Red clover.** Popular, but unproven benefits for mild menopausal symptoms.
- **Ginseng.** Some evidence it improves sleep and mood, but not helpful for hot flashes. There are reports of possible heart damage over time.
- **St. John's wort.** Clearly helps mild depression and mood swings. Some believe combining this with black cohosh may be especially helpful.
- **Dong Quai.** Used in traditional Chinese medicine. Modern studies show no benefit for hot flashes, and it may cause cancer when used long term.
- **Evening primrose oil.** One controlled study evaluating use for menopausal symptoms showed a mild decrease in the intensity of hot flashes, but not in their frequency.[2]

Soy products deserve an honorable mention. The phytoestrogens in soy do have some estrogen-like effect in the body, and modest evidence indicates they may improve mild menopausal symptoms in some women. A greater concern is that there's no standardized quality control in the production of soy supplements, so there's no clear recommendation on what dose is safe or effective.

Because of the estrogen activity of phytoestrogens, there is some concern about their risk for increasing breast cancer or uterine cancer. There is very limited data and no clear answer either way. But you absolutely cannot assume these products are safer than prescription estradiol. I believe a woman who still has a uterus and is taking regular phytoestrogen supplements should also consider natural progesterone or have yearly pelvic ultrasounds and get regular mammograms.

We cover more information on supplements in general in chapter 17.

NONHORMONAL MEDICATIONS

Several nonhormonal prescription options may help those women who choose to avoid hormone therapy. What might work for you is dependent on what symptoms are most troublesome to you. No one medication is likely to "fix" all your symptoms.

SSRI and SNRI antidepressants will often decrease hot flashes. Medications where studies document this improvement include Prozac (fluoxetine), Zoloft (sertraline), Cymbalta (duloxetine), and Effexor (venlafaxine). Brisdelle (a variety of paroxetine) is now FDA approved for treating menopausal hot flashes. These medications affect the neurotransmitters serotonin and/or norepinephrine that are involved in triggering hot flashes and may be especially helpful if you're also struggling with depression.

Osphena is the first non-estrogen oral medication specifically approved to treat painful vaginal dryness affecting intercourse. It is a selective estrogen-receptor modulator (SERM) that works similarly to estrogen in some body tissues, including the vagina, and helps vaginal tissue become more elastic and moist. It doesn't help hot flashes and may slightly increase your risk of uterine cancer.

We'll talk more about loss of bone mineral (which is the risk of osteoporosis) in chapter 12 and more about mental and emotional challenges in chapter 20.

Other Symptoms

A few other symptoms deserve comment. You may find yourself facing these symptoms when you enter menopause:

+ **Trouble sleeping.** Hot flashes at night—night sweats—may seriously disturb your ability to get adequate rest even if you aren't aware of waking up. So can anxiety, frequent urination, or aches and pains. Sleeping in a cool room, sleeping with layers (so you can throw some off if needed), and learning healthy ways to manage stress will improve your sleep. Medications that lessen hot flashes usually help you sleep better also.

+ **Vaginal dryness.** Most women, either at the time of menopause or years later, experience this. Over-the-counter lubricants such as Astroglide or Replens can help your general comfort level and make intercourse more pleasant. If you choose to try estrogen, vaginal estradiol is especially helpful. And the non-estrogen Osphena is another prescription option (see above).

+ **Pelvic organ prolapse.** Loosening of the vaginal tissues and muscles may allow the bladder, cervix, uterus, and/or rectum to "fall down" into the vaginal area. This may cause pressure, discomfort, urinary problems, and other symptoms. Estrogen may only help a little. Kegel exercises are helpful for some women.[3] Consider a physical therapist who specializes in the pelvic muscles. Some women need surgery to try and restore the pelvic anatomy to near normal.

+ **Libido.** Hormone changes are only part of the reason many women experience decreased sexual desire after menopause (though some experience increased libido). Physical exercise, good sleep, stress management, and working on your marriage relationship will help. Some women find estrogen therapy helpful because intercourse is no longer painful. (We'll cover more of this in chapter 21.)

+ **Memory.** Whether or not estrogen and menopausal hormonal changes affect thinking and memory is somewhat controversial. There's more on "menopause brain" in chapter 20.

LIFESTYLE MEASURES

Imagine a pill that would help you sleep better, increase your energy, decrease your hot flashes, improve your mood and memory, and make you feel happier. This same pill would help you lose weight, look and feel younger, live longer, and decrease your risk for depression, dementia, diabetes, heart disease, stroke, and osteoporosis. It would decrease your risk of disability and of ending up in a nursing home. It would improve almost every measure of quality of life. And it's totally free. Would you take that pill? I know I would.

The truth is, you already have this pill! And it's in your closet right now—in the form of a pair of walking shoes. Every one of those elements I described above has been proven over and over again to be a benefit of regular physical exercise, especially for women going through menopause. It truly is the magic potion.

If you're like me, you'll say, "Sure, I know that. I just don't want to do it." Regular exercise is the area of my physical health that I struggle with the most. But that doesn't mean you and I shouldn't keep on trying. Find someone to exercise with. Find an activity you enjoy. And just do it.

Eating a diet largely made up of fruits, vegetables, and lean protein will also serve you well. In this season of life, your body is less able to handle processed food, especially processed carbohydrates, than it was previously. Eating a healthy diet will help you feel more energetic and help you control the weight gain many menopausal women struggle with.

The North American Menopause Society, available at www.meno pause.org, provides a lot of patient-friendly resources you may find helpful. And hey, if you're still having hot flashes, why not think of them as power surges instead?

A Few Questions

Q: How long will I have menopausal symptoms?

A: Some women only have hot flashes for two to three years, while about 15 percent of women continue to have symptoms indefinitely. If you're taking hormone medication, try stopping it briefly every year or two to see if your symptoms return. If they do, keep taking hormones unless your doctor discovers other problems that mean you should stop. As women progress past the menopause transition, they often need a lower amount of estrogen to manage their symptoms, and you may be able to decrease your dose over time.

Q: If I take estrogen, how much should I take?

A: Some companies or practitioners have made a lot of money selling blood or saliva tests to "personalize" hormone therapy. There's no evidence that such testing is helpful. If you have symptoms that are consistent with a lack of estrogen, blood tests that confirm that you're at least perimenopausal (near menopause) and rule out other medical issues are appropriate. From that point on, therapy should be guided by your symptoms. In rare cases, blood tests that confirm that you're absorbing estradiol may be helpful, but not in order to adjust the dose.

Q: Does my attitude on aging affect my health during menopause?

A: Yes! Several studies have documented that a positive attitude toward aging will allow you to live longer with less illness and disability—7.5 years longer, according to one study.[4] Treasure the productivity, wisdom, and perspective your stage in life affords.

Section 2

LONG-TERM
HEALTH

Chapter 9

EAT TO LIVE

YOU CAN ONLY get by without food for a matter of days or weeks, although the way some people go after it, you'd think they could only survive without it for a matter of minutes. People in some cultures spend the majority of their time searching for and preparing it—and most of their limited finances buying it. Books about it are some of the best sellers around. It's the stuff of satisfaction, celebration, community, and, most of all, *life*.

You really are what you eat, and in several ways. Food is a big part of who we are. It means nutrition. But it also means a whole lot more. It can relieve stress or cause it. It can ease suffering or increase your risk of disease. Unhealthy eating has been associated with a whole host of problems. In no particular order, the list includes heart disease, cancer, diabetes, stroke, high blood pressure, immune problems, bowel problems, acne, painful joints, eczema, mood disorders, fatigue, kidney disease, obesity, PMS, forgetfulness, and Alzheimer's disease. And that's just a short list. Some of these problems have other causes also, but your diet is at least one significant factor in them all.

And then there are the social, ethical, and political aspects of food. The many people in our world, and even in our own neighborhoods, who are hungry or starving contrasts bluntly with the many who are overfed. Food stamps, school lunches, food banks, government farm policy, FDA regulations—food is a big deal.

Healthy eating doesn't have to be restrictive, difficult, complicated, expensive, or socially exploitative. There are simple principles that will help you enjoy the health that good eating can afford while avoiding the pitfalls of either excess or deprivation. Food can be a true friend rather than a frenemy.

FOOD CAN MAKE YOU SICK OR HEALTHY

There is a huge amount of research on food and disease. It's so vast that one could make a career out of compiling, organizing, and categorizing the thousands of scientific studies, books, programs, diets, Internet resources, and more that exist. But you don't have time for that. So in order to relay the vast array of all this science more simply, here are some focused food facts that matter to your health. (Don't get hung up here; we'll apply these items to your diet a little later.)

Food matters.

Scientists estimate that at the last turn of the century, in the year 2000, the combination of a poor diet and lack of physical activity was the underlying cause in over 16 percent of deaths in the United States,[1] and many believe the true number may be even higher. Unhealthy eating can kill you! Much of the difference in death and disease rates in different cultures can be explained by eating patterns.

Processed matters.

Processed means foods that are not natural or not as close to their natural state as possible. Many processed foods contain added salt, sugar, flavorings, preservatives, or other chemicals. Refined grains fall into this category because of how differently they react in the body compared with whole (natural) grains. Processed foods usually have a longer shelf life, usually come in a package, and are often highly flavored. These foods are implicated in cancer, heart disease, obesity, Alzheimer's, diabetes, and autoimmune diseases. And these foods make up the majority of what most Americans eat! This is probably the single most important dietary factor of all.

> **Health Tip**
>
> *If it's in a box or a package, it's probably processed. Decrease the processed foods in your diet, and you'll be healthier.*

Sugar matters.

Regardless of weight, added sugar appears to be a significant factor in heart disease,[2] mental health,[3] and other illnesses. Insulin resistance (more than eating too much sugar) has been associated with diabetes, reproductive problems, and much more.

Fats matter.

Saturated fats, unsaturated fats, trans fats—all of it can be confusing. Your body needs some fat intake regularly. The data blaming trans fats for a number of health risks is very convincing. The data on saturated fat and red meat is less overwhelming, while omega-3 fatty acids (i.e., fish oil) are clearly beneficial in many ways.

Fiber matters.

Fiber comes from natural fruits, vegetables, legumes such as beans and peas, and whole grains. Too little fiber has been associated with heart disease, obesity, some cancers, intestinal problems, and diabetes.[4]

Inflammation matters.

Chronic inflammation is an underlying factor in many illnesses, including cardiovascular disease, immune disorders, cancer, Alzheimer's disease, and more. Dietary factors, including the glycemic index (see the next section), type of fats ingested, and other phytonutrients affect inflammation significantly—some positively, some negatively.[5]

Organic matters just a little.

Organic foods are free (or mostly free) of pesticides, insecticides, fertilizers, and the like. There is no clear evidence they are more nutritious. And in general, the level of chemicals in nonorganic produce is low, probably low enough to have little or no effect on health for most people. If you want to go organic but don't have the extra money to buy organic for everything, consider the Dirty Dozen a top priority. (The Dirty Dozen is a list compiled by the Environmental Working Group of the fruits and vegetables containing the highest levels of pesticides. The list is revised each year and can be found at www.ewg.org/food news/dirty_dozen_list.php.)

Does all of this sound complicated? It really isn't. Many of these principles overlap. For example, foods that are processed are the same foods that promote inflammation, contain the least fiber, and contain the most sugar, unhealthy fats, and artificial chemicals.

A word on the glycemic index (GI) is appropriate. This is a score given to each food indicating how much and how rapidly it increases your blood sugar. Moving to foods that have a lower glycemic index is likely to decrease your blood sugar and insulin levels and may decrease inflammation in your body. Following a diet based on the GI can be somewhat complicated, and most people can develop a much simpler healthy eating plan than scoring the GI of every food they eat. You can learn more about the glycemic index at www.glycemicindex.com.

Nutrition Data has provided a very useful source of information on specific foods at www.nutritiondata.self.com. Simply enter the food you're interested in, and you'll get a ton of information including the nutrient makeup, glycemic load, inflammatory index, and more.

If you want to make one dietary change that will result in better health, make the move to less-processed foods. This week choose one processed food you normally eat and choose a less-processed alternative. That might be choosing fajita-style chicken instead of lunch meat, frozen stir-fry instead of a TV dinner, or instant oatmeal instead of boxed breakfast cereal. It doesn't have to be fresh off the produce truck to be healthier; just choose something one step less processed.

Health Tip

Make the move to less-processed food. Each week, swap out one processed food for one less processed until at least 80 percent of your food is less processed.

And then next week swap out another processed food. Keep doing this until at least 80 percent of your food is less processed, and you'll have a dramatically healthier diet.

And by the way, the chemicals in processed foods are much more dangerous to your health than the comparatively small amount of chemicals in nonorganic produce. A hot dog or a nonorganic apple? There's no contest.

It's Not About the Diet

"Mirror, mirror, on the wall, what's the healthiest diet of them all?" Truthfully, no diet at all! I think *diet* is a dirty word. It implies restricting what you eat while you're on the diet and then going back to how you were eating before when you go off the diet. It's much wiser to make smaller lifestyle changes that you can stay with long term. That's the only diet that will improve your long-term health. We're looking for both simple *and* healthy.

Many diets have been developed based on extremes: low-fat, no-carb, raw only, gluten-free, paleo, organic, detox. Some of you will cry "Foul!" here, because you follow one of those plans and believe it has helped you. Good for you! Some people need an extraordinarily restricted diet because of a specific health problem. But it's just that: extraordinary.

Most people simply need a wide variety of healthy foods on a regular basis. Researchers summarized all the scientific evidence on diet and health like this: "A diet of minimally processed foods close to nature, predominantly plants, is decisively associated with health promotion and disease prevention."[6] You don't need to spend a lot of money on expensive food and supplements or completely deprive yourself of your favorite treats. If 80 to 90 percent of your food is healthy, it's OK to enjoy something "forbidden" once in a while.

I can't generally recommend most of the popular diets out there for several reasons. A restrictive diet (such as a no-carb diet) almost always eliminates many of the good, healthy foods your body needs. And it's extremely difficult to stick with a restrictive diet over the long term. If you feel the need to cleanse your body after a stressful holiday season or absolutely must lose ten pounds in two weeks, go on a restrictive diet temporarily. But that won't improve your long-term health at all.

A few specifics on diets:

+ **No-carb diet.** Eating this way puts a tremendous burden on your kidneys and your gastrointestinal system. A strict no-carb diet severely limits fruits and vegetables, which are full of healthy phytonutrients. Many people lose weight if they follow this diet regularly, but it's not healthy long term. (This applies to severely low-carb diets, like Atkins or South Beach, as well.)

+ **Low-fat diet.** Most Americans could do well to eat less fat, especially trans fats. However, many products labeled low fat are not very healthy. They're often processed and contain plenty of sugar, artificial flavoring, or other bad stuff. You need regular amounts of good fats, such as olive oil or fish oil. There are much better things to focus on than limiting fat in your diet.

+ **Gluten-free diet.** Unless someone has Celiac disease (a specific illness where the GI system can't process gluten), going completely gluten-free isn't likely to be helpful. A gluten-free diet eliminates much of the healthy vitamins and fiber in whole grains. However, cutting back significantly on baked goods, pasta, and the like will decrease the processed carbohydrates you eat, and that's a very good thing.

+ **Paleo diet.** There are some good things about the Paleo diet, such as limiting processed foods. But the heavy emphasis on meat is inconsistent with what your body needs for good health. There's no evidence that eliminating whole grains and dairy from your diet will be beneficial to your long-term health.

+ **Organic, detox, or raw-only diets.** There's nothing wrong with choosing organic produce as long as you follow the other healthy eating principles outlined below. A raw-only diet is extremely restrictive, and there's no evidence it's beneficial to your health. And if you choose some type of detox diet, just make sure it's only for a short time.

So, what type of eating plan is healthiest? If I have to recommend a diet, the Mediterranean diet definitely comes out on top. This eating plan focuses on fresh food, olive oil, and some fish. Moderate amounts of red wine are commonly included. Baked goods and red meat are eaten sparingly if at all. And interestingly, simply adding olive oil or nuts to your diet can make a significant improvement in your health, even if you don't specifically follow the other aspects of this diet.[7] You don't have to follow a specific, written Mediterranean diet plan to get the benefits. Most of the principles are the same as what is outlined here.

YOUR HEALTHY EATING PLAN

My friend and wellness expert Kathrine Lee[8] likens each of your body's cells to a baby bird with a wide-open mouth, crying, "Feed me! Feed me!" If you dump enough dirt on the baby birds, they'll be quiet for a time. But if the dirt doesn't kill them, they'll soon start crying for food again. So it is with you. Filling your stomach with empty calories will stop your hunger pains—for now. But if your cells aren't getting the nutrition they need, they'll soon start crying for food again. And those cells crave a lot more than just calories.

So, how do we satisfy those starving-baby-bird cells? Here's how.

Water

Water is for more than just showers. It is also the best beverage to drink. If you don't like water, try switching gradually. Try flavored water, such as Crystal Light, as a transition; it's certainly better than soda. Or try a cucumber slice, lemon, or strawberry in a glass of ice water.

What kind of water is best? The kind you will drink! Some bottled water is no different from tap water. If you don't care for the taste in your water supply or if you wish to decrease the small amount of chemicals in most commercial water, purchase an inexpensive water filter to put on your kitchen tap or refrigerator water supply. There is no evidence that an expensive water system (such as reverse osmosis, ionized, or pH balanced) will make a significant improvement in your health. If you live in an area with a commercial water supply, there's no excuse to drink sodas because you don't want to purchase a water-filtration system!

Sugar-sweetened beverages and fruit juice raise your blood sugar quickly, increasing insulin, fat production, and inflammation throughout your body. When your blood sugar crashes, you're hungry again—for more sugar. It's the ulti-mate "dump" on those baby-bird-hungry cells. An occasional cup of fruit juice is OK, but not as your primary source of liquid.

> **Dr. Carol Says ...**
>
> *"What kind of water is best? The kind you will drink!"*

Sports drinks and energy drinks generally contain significant amounts of sugar, caffeine, artificial sweeteners, and/or other artificial ingredients. If you're struggling with vomiting or diarrhea or are exercising strenuously and need electrolytes, these drinks may be helpful. Otherwise these are best left alone.

Fruits and vegetables

There is no better way to pack more nutrients into your diet and satisfy those baby-bird-hungry cells than to choose food that grows from the ground or falls from a tree. The natural fiber is also great for your cardiovascular and digestive systems.

When choosing fruits and veggies, remember:

+ **Fresher is better.** Produce that's in season is likely fresher and less expensive than that which isn't. Try a farmer's market. Remember that organic may not be worth the extra money. If you want to buy organic for only the worst offenders, check the list of the Dirty Dozen fruits and veg-gies at www.ewg.org/foodnews/dirty_dozen_list.php.
+ **Fresh first, frozen second, canned third.** Fruits and veggies are generally frozen at near-peak ripeness, and little if any

nutrition is lost. They may contain more nutrition than fresh produce picked too green or languishing on the shelf.

Canning adds a level of processing to produce that decreases its nutritional value. Eating canned? Choose fruit in light syrup or natural juice to limit the sugar, and rinse canned vegetables before using to remove some of the added sodium.

+ **Darker, brighter, and more colorful means more nutritious.** Think dark green, bright yellow, deep purple, bright red. Those natural foods that pack the most nutrition per serving include red and purple berries and dark greens like kale, collards, and spinach.

+ **Add more.** Adding fruits and vegetables to your diet can be one of the healthiest changes you can make. You need several servings each day.

Lean protein

Going vegetarian can be a healthy way of eating. Beans, legumes, and nuts have great fiber and protein. Soaking beans overnight and then cooking them long and slow will lessen the flatulence factor. Sometimes taking an enzyme, such as Beano, will lessen any bloating or gas.

If you eat meat, here are some things to remember:

+ **Less red.** Research demonstrates many reasons to limit red meat. Eating more red meat may cause an increased risk of heart disease and certain cancers. One or two servings of lean red meat per week isn't likely to increase your health risks significantly.

+ **Prepare leanly.** Fried food appears to be one big reason why the South is known as the stroke belt. Grilling at high temperatures is also dangerous, producing cancer-causing heterocyclic amines (HCAs). Baking, broiling, and slow-cooking are healthiest.

+ **Say no to processed.** This may be the most important choice of all. Eating processed meat (such as hot dogs, bacon, ham, and sausage) increases your risk of premature death more than most other dietary factors.[9]

+ **Rethink dairy.** Most people can safely use moderate
amounts of dairy products as a healthy part of their diet.
Milk and milk products can be a great source of calcium and
protein. Controversy exists over whether reduced-fat or whole
milk is preferable.
+ **Use caution with cheese.** Some vegetarians simply substitute cheese for meat. That's not healthy! Cheese packs
too much fat to be a wise primary source of protein; use it
occasionally.
+ **Consider organic.** There is significant concern about additives in even unprocessed meat, such as antibiotics or other
chemicals used in the care of animals, fish, or poultry from
which the meat in our food supply comes. There's something
to be said for free-range, wild, or grass-fed when it comes to
meat. Choosing organic meat makes even more sense than
it does for produce. However, processed or high-fat meat is
a much greater danger to your health than nonorganic meat
ever would be.

Fats

Second to water, your brain is mostly fat. The walls of your body's
cells are made of fats. You need some healthy fats every day. The trick
is to separate the good, the bad, and the ugly.

+ **The good.** You need the polyunsaturated fats that are found
in olive oil, nuts, and avocados for brain function and more.
Consider switching to olive oil for daily use. This step alone
has been found to improve longevity and cardiovascular
health.[10]
+ **The ugly.** Trans fats, which are found in many baked and
fried foods, margarine, and desserts, clog up your cardiovascular system. Read food labels, and keep your daily intake of
trans fats to less than 1 gram.
+ **The bad.** Almost everything else. They add calories while
adding minimal nutrition and may increase cholesterol. Use
in limited amounts.

Whole grains

The difference between eating processed, refined flour products and whole grains is as different as night and day, at least as far as your health is concerned. Processed refined flour, found in most baked goods, cereals, pasta, and snacks, has been linked to depression, cardiovascular disease, diabetes, and more. There is something very unhealthy about refined wheat flour.

Whole grains, however, are an excellent source of fiber, protein, B vitamins, and other essential nutrients. Two new high-quality studies demonstrate that eating more whole grains decreases cardiovascular disease and death from all causes.[11] The biggest single factor explaining the positive effect on health was the amount of bran eaten. Other research also correlates eating whole grains with a decreased risk of diabetes.

Steel-cut oats probably have the best reputation of all, but other whole grains can be healthy also, such as barley, whole wheat, whole-grain rice, and millet. Whole-grain bread and cereal can be part of a healthy diet.

What Should You Eat?

In summary at least 80 percent of your diet should be:

+ A variety of colorful fruits and vegetables
+ Lean protein, such as beans, fish, and poultry
+ Healthy fats, such as olive oil, nuts, and avocados
+ Unprocessed whole grains
+ Water

The hamburger or hot dog, the bacon, the pasta with meat sauce, the croissant, the TV dinner, the Oreo cookie, the ice cream—if you keep all of these to the less than 20 percent of your diet that is discretionary, you'll probably do just fine.

And finally, slow down! It takes your brain twenty minutes to register what you've eaten. Take a small portion, and savor every bite. If you're still hungry a while later, take another portion. Food was meant to be enjoyed!

For almost all of us, food will be there again tomorrow. Jesus asked us to pray, "Give us today our daily bread" (Matt. 6:11). Fresher, cleaner, simpler—and just enough for today.

A Few Questions

Q: Can a vegetarian or vegan diet be healthy?

A: Absolutely. I've been a vegetarian during significant portions of my life. However, avoiding meat or animal products entirely does not, in itself, make a diet healthy. Some vegetarians eat large amounts of processed foods and refined carbohydrates with all the chemicals included or use fatty cheese as a primary source of protein, and that's not healthy. The principles in this chapter apply whether you choose to be a vegetarian or not.

Q: What's the story on artificial sweeteners?

A: There's been a lot of debate here. My summary of the evidence is that artificial sweeteners carry significant health risks, may be addictive, and definitely increase food cravings. For most people, small amounts of sugar are probably safer. If you must use artificial sweeteners, Stevia is probably safest, followed by Splenda.

Q: What do you believe about coffee and tea?

A: A variety of research favors coffee and tea as being healthy for most people, though not all studies agree. Green tea, especially, has well-documented health benefits. But beware of the additives! Fat, sugar, and artificial flavorings add up fast. A mocha latte should be an occasional dessert, not a regular morning pick-me-up.

Chapter 10

MANAGING YOUR WEIGHT

MY HUSBAND, AL, is a wonderful success story. When we first met, he was a smoker, enjoyed the typical unhealthy American diet, and was quite overweight. He successfully stopped smoking when we got married but gained even more weight after that. His obesity was affecting his health, his sleep, his self-esteem, and our relationship.

But that's not the end of the story. I'll always remember the visit when his doctor asked me, "What diet do you have him on? He's doing great!" At that time he had lost about sixty pounds, and he's lost more since. And it's been without any diet, supplements, pills, surgery, or other gimmicks. He's never missed a meal, and we still keep ice cream in the freezer. He's ninety pounds lighter now and healthier than ever.

Al didn't lose his weight in a week, a month, or even a year. It's been slow and steady, but it's been healthy and permanent. He's never felt deprived.

I love sharing his story because if he can do it, you can do it too. I know you can lose weight if you need to. In this chapter, I'll share with you what I call "Dr. Carol's No-Pills, No-Supplements, No-Surgery, Guaranteed Way to Lose Any Amount of Weight."

WHAT'S YOUR MOTIVATION?

"I don't want to have to lose weight to get a man. I want a man to love me just the way I am!" And the tears rolled freely.

Nancy was a young second-grade teacher, unhappily single, and already experiencing physical problems as a result of being seriously overweight. But the emotional complications affected her even more. She asked my opinion about weight-loss surgery. More than the risks of surgery, she was most concerned that a thinner body might make her attractive to a man who would want her for the wrong reasons.

If you struggle with your weight, you know how hard it can be. And that struggle is about much more than a number on the scale. You already know obesity increases disability and shortens life expectancy.[1]

It's also very expensive—in health-care costs,[2] in relationships, in dollars spent trying to lose weight, and more. In the United States alone, the diet-control and weight-loss market is worth $61 billion per year.[3]

Yes, you will almost certainly have more energy and be physically healthier if you carry around less body fat. Losing weight to feel better and be healthier is a worthy goal in itself. So it's natural to think, *If only I were thinner, I would be happy.* But simply losing weight won't automatically bring you happiness.

If you want to lose weight, ask yourself why. Are you sick and tired of feeling sick and tired, and are you committed to making the necessary lifestyle changes so that you can feel better? Are you owning the fact that being overweight is affecting the people closest to you? Are you willing to do the work necessary so that you're able to give your best to your loved ones? Do you feel God creating the desire in your heart to become a better advertisement for His kingdom by being physically healthier?

Changing lifestyle behaviors on the outside is important. But it's even more important to face what is going on inside your heart. Owning your *why* will make all the other necessary changes easier.

If you could wave a magic wand and suddenly be at your ideal body weight, would you do so? I know individuals who have lost tremendous amounts of weight and are miserable. You don't want to be one of them. Make sure you deal with whatever is weighing you down on the inside along with your physical weight.

THE HUNGERS WE FACE

Ann knew she was experiencing some health problems as a result of being seriously overweight. She had very little energy, her knees hurt all the time, her menstrual cycle was messed up, and her cholesterol level was dangerously high. She knew she needed to lose weight, and the first step in doing so was eating healthier. But she was finding that very difficult. She sat on the exam table and told me, "I'm an emotional eater. It's the way I handle stress."

At least Ann realizes there is a difference between physical hunger and emotional hunger. We have many different needs. When one of those needs isn't met, we feel hungry. But it may not be a hunger for food.

Sometimes hunger signals a physical need for nutrition—your body needs fuel. But that same feeling may also signal a need for many other things. Each of us has our "go-to" means of trying to satisfy that feeling of hunger when it comes. You may reach for food. Someone else may reach for a cigarette, find someone to yell at, or go for a run.

Feeding emotional hunger with physical food may lessen the "Feed me!" voice screaming in your brain, but only for a little while. When the underlying need hasn't been met, the mental demand for food only gets louder once again, and a vicious cycle can develop. You feel hungry, so you eat food (perhaps unhealthy food); the underlying hunger isn't met, so you feel even more hungry—as well as guilty—so you eat more food; then you feel more hungry and more guilty. The cycle goes on and on.

Health Tip

To lose weight, first deal with what's eating you.

Using physical food to meet an emotional need often leads to other side effects, including frustration, sluggish mental thinking, obesity, and guilt. Kathrine Lee likes to say, "It's not what you're eating; it's what's eating you." Understanding and meeting the different needs you have with appropriate nourishment will impact your health and happiness in many ways. The key is thinking through what kind of nourishment you need most.

If you normally reach for food to try to quiet any hunger you feel, it may take some thinking and self-study to understand what your body and mind is asking for. Here are some of the hungers we can misinterpret as a need for food:

+ **Thirst.** Many people feel they're hungry when they're really thirsty. A cold glass of ice water (flavored, if necessary) may satisfy what your brain is screaming for better than food. Dehydration can lead to irritability, headaches, fatigue, and just plain feeling bad. And alcohol, carbonated beverages, or caffeine won't do the trick.

+ **Lack of energy.** How many times have you reached for food as a pick-me-up during the late-morning, late-afternoon, or late-evening hours when you feel your mind and body drag? Eating processed food often gives a quick energy surge from the rapid increase in blood sugar, only to result in a crash later on. And turning to caffeine or more sugar only makes things worse.

+ **Fatigue.** I often used food to stay awake while studying for exams in medical school or during a long, cross-country car trip. But what my brain and body really needed was sleep. Food doesn't resolve the tiredness; only rest will do that.

+ **Stress relief.** Eating is something to do, something in your hands, something in your mouth. You grab food when your spouse yells at you, the collection agency calls, or your child comes home with a bad report card. Food is an easy "go-to" for stress relief—or anger or fear or any other strong emotion—but provides a very poor outcome. And the stress doesn't go away.

+ **Boredom.** Food can provide something sweet, something salty, something crunchy, something to graze on when you aren't doing anything else. You munch on food while watching TV, working on a boring project, or waiting for someone else to show up. Yes, it keeps your hands and mouth busy, but your body will pay the price later.

+ **Loneliness.** Hungry for some tender loving care? What you really need may be a hug. When no one is around to provide one, food can become a hopeful substitute. It doesn't fill the nagging need in your soul for human connection, however. It only temporarily covers it up.

+ **Unhappiness.** It's a vicious cycle. You eat for comfort, to feel better, to feel anything but unhappy. Then you feel worse because you're overweight or unhealthy or feel guilty. And then you eat more to feel comforted again, so the cycle continues.

As an unhappy young woman I used food to soothe my unhappiness for a number of years. People who know me now are surprised when I tell them that. During those years I was heavier than I needed to be. I was also extremely unhappy and used food as a means to cope. For me, when I learned how to be happy, the food took care of itself.

Your journey may be easier or harder than mine. But facing the hungers in your soul will make all the difference.

Ultimately, there's a primary hunger in the soul that no food, no physical substance, and no human being can satisfy. The reality of hunger—that desire—is God's idea. Otherwise we would never search for what we need most. It's when we try and meet those deepest needs with material things that we get into trouble.

MY PLAN FOR YOU

Now for the nitty-gritty work of actually shedding those pounds. There are certainly some medical illnesses that prevent some people from losing weight. I see some of these people in my office. But the most common illness causing obesity is an unwillingness to put down the fork and put on walking shoes.

> ### Dr. Carol Says...
>
> *"The most common cause of obesity is an unwillingness to put down the fork and put on walking shoes."*

I know it's not politically correct to say that. There is so much talk about communities not having safe places to exercise, neighborhoods not having grocery stores that provide healthy food, and cheap prices and marketing of processed foods that make healthy food less appealing. Of course we need to improve public policies and make it easier for people to make healthier choices.

But none of that is an excuse. Do you really want to give the government the responsibility for deciding how much you weigh? Your genes, your environment, and your financial status may make certain choices easier or harder for you—but they're still *your* choices. *You* get to decide what to eat today and how much you want to weigh next year or ten years from now.

Promoting slow and steady weight loss isn't very sexy. It won't get you on TV. It won't make you a lot of money. But it's almost always healthiest. Quick weight loss feels great, but weight that comes off quickly almost always goes back on just as quickly. Most people should aim to lose one to five pounds per week. That goal is attainable through lifestyle changes. And those changes should be ones you can stay with long-term.

That may not sound like an effective strategy. But just think: if you lose just two pounds a week and keep it up for one year, you'll be 100 pounds lighter this time next year! The key is longevity—finding small changes you can make permanent.

At the beginning of this chapter I promised to share with you "Dr. Carol's No-Pills, No-Supplements, No-Surgery, Guaranteed Way to Lose Any Amount of Weight." Here's the ten-point plan guaranteed to help you do just that.

1. *Know that you are more than your body weight.* Your happiness, your relationships, and your spiritual life are all more important than your BMI (body mass index).[4] Keep things in perspective. Actively invest in other parts of your life. Have fun, keep up personal relationships, learn new things, and commit to your spiritual growth.

   ### Health Tip

   Most people should aim to lose one to five pounds per week. That goal is attainable and can result in permanent weight loss.

2. *Toss the extra baggage.* Remember that it's not what you're eating; it's what's eating you. Deal with the emotional, mental, relational, or spiritual baggage that is weighing you down. When you do, food will become a much smaller problem.

3. *Keep it natural.* Increase the natural foods in your diet, especially fruits and vegetables. Include some unprocessed protein every day, ideally at every meal. Look for processed food in your diet, and each week change out one processed food for one closer to its natural state until 80 to 90 percent of your food is unprocessed.

4. *Give your brain a chance.* It takes about twenty minutes for your brain to process how much food you've eaten. At each meal, prepare a moderate amount of

food. Place a smaller-than-usual portion on your plate, and eat it slowly. When you're finished with that portion, discipline yourself to wait twenty minutes. Then ask yourself, "Am I truly still hungry?" If you are, take another small portion and eat it slowly.

5. *Address the stress.* If you use food to manage stress, boredom, or loneliness, find other ways to manage those problems. Find habits you can develop in place of snacking, such as calling a friend, drinking some water, or taking a five-minute walk. And guard your sleep; adequate rest will help you lose weight.

6. *Know that deprivation doesn't work.* Eventually you will relapse if you try to completely deprive yourself of your favorite foods. If 90 percent of your diet is healthy, it's OK to enjoy some treats now and then. (If you're trying hard to lose weight, you may need this 90/10 rule instead of the 80/20 rule mentioned in the previous chapter.)

7. *Don't do it alone.* Accountability to a spouse, a good friend, or a professional will make you much more successful. Tell them what you want to accomplish and what you need from them to help you succeed. Get over your pride, and accept their encouragement, feedback, and support.

8. *Get moving.* The power of exercise added to a healthy diet will take away more pounds than you realize. It doesn't matter very much what you do; just move more today than you did yesterday. Find a girlfriend to go walking with—even inside the mall if outside is difficult. Join an exercise class or swim team if you want to. Get a treadmill and walk while watching TV or listening to podcasts.

9. *Remember that small changes add up.* You don't have to get back to an ideal body weight to start experiencing significant health benefits. Losing just 10 percent of your body weight will create a major shift in

your sense of well-being, your hormonal and metabolic system, and your long-term risk of disease and death. (I tell my patients to make losing 10 percent their initial goal.)

10. *Take it one day at a time.* As with any lifestyle change, losing weight is a process. Small changes today add up to big results over time. If you "fall off the wagon," get back up tomorrow and try again. That's normal! Each time you make a mistake, look at what might have gone wrong, and use what you learn to set yourself up for success next time.

Lifestyle change feels like a slow way to lose weight. The long-term benefits, however, make it the only way to go for almost everyone, and it's the best method to assure your weight loss will last for a long time.

Another word about processed foods: they're bad for your health in general, but they're like poison if you need to lose weight. Baked goods, sugary cereals, processed meats, TV dinners, convenience snacks, and most desserts will sabotage your weight-loss goals almost every time. The added flavorings, sugar, and salt make these foods "hyperpalatable"; they create cravings in your brain for more, like a drug addiction. Most include refined carbohydrates, which quickly raise blood sugar, increase insulin levels, and are easily converted to body fat.

If there's an ideal eating plan for losing weight, it's this: keep it natural! Go for my recommendation to replace one processed food with a less-processed alternative each week until at least 80 percent of your food is more natural. Try substituting fish sticks with baked tilapia, chips with apple slices and peanut butter, or sugary cereal with oatmeal. That's exactly how my husband lost ninety pounds without missing a meal or going on a diet.

PRODUCTS, PROGRAMS, AND SURGERY

I don't know anyone who seriously struggles with weight who hasn't thought about—and probably tried—a number of weight-loss products. Notice the shelf space devoted to these products in any grocery store or pharmacy. It's big business. But do they work?

Spending hundreds of dollars each month on a program like Nutrisystem, Medifast, or ViSalus can provide you with a lot of motivation toward a healthier lifestyle. These programs focus on meal replacement, and research shows they can result in significant weight loss. But there's no magic. You can accomplish the same thing with a plant-based diet and by limiting processed foods, using portion control—and having some discipline.

Now for some bad news: supplements and products claiming to melt away pounds *without any change in lifestyle* are either dangerous or worthless. That's a strong statement, but I can't find even one that comes with a reassuring measure of scientific support. Whenever you see or hear about such a product, demand to see double-blind, placebo-controlled research before you spend your hard-earned money for something that doesn't work. Don't be a sucker.

Along with lifestyle change, research demonstrating the benefits of any available supplements is mixed. Most studies of reasonable quality show little or no benefit. Some supplements, such as ephedra or bitter orange, are downright dangerous because of their stimulant effects. There is some limited encouraging research that adding green tea extract or green coffee extract to healthy dietary changes may help with weight loss.

A few prescription medications may be helpful for some women battling obesity. Metformin isn't a weight-loss medication, but for women with diabetes or prediabetes it may be very helpful in losing weight. The Fen-Phen disaster has appropriately caused great caution among pharmaceutical companies and regulators to make certain that the risks of any approved medication don't outweigh the weight-loss benefits. A few prescription medications have been approved to treat obesity by curbing your appetite, though each has potential side effects. Have a long discussion with your doctor before using any of these medications.

What about weight-loss surgery? Available surgical options include gastric bypass, lap-band placement, and sleeve gastrectomy. All are likely to result in significant weight loss and lower your risk of diabetes and other obesity-related illnesses. But none of the surgical options are risk free. I know people who have done well after weight-loss surgery and others who have experienced serious complications. Even more important, weight loss achieved this way doesn't automatically make you happier. If you do choose surgery, it's even more important to address the lifestyle, emotional, relationship, or spiritual issues you may also be facing.

If you choose meal-replacement programs, supplements, prescription medication, or surgery, I encourage you to view those methods as an additional boost to the lifestyle changes you are committed to making. You, your loved ones, and others you will help throughout your life are worth your efforts to become healthier.

DOES GOD CARE IF YOU'RE FAT?

Here we get to the issue of shame. Standing naked before your husband or your God can feel terrifying. Being or feeling overweight may be only one of the aspects of shame you're dealing with, and it starts early, with messages from parents, peers, media, and culture.

How does God feel about your weight? First of all, remember that God won't check your BMI on your way into heaven. There are no scales at the foot of the cross or at the pearly gates. How God feels about you is based on your faith in Jesus, not the number of pounds you weigh.

God also understands you better than you understand yourself. He understands the physical or emotional pain you may feel, and He hurts when you hurt. He knows your weaknesses and understands the struggles you've been through trying to lose weight. He's not a taskmaster who is forcing you to do something. He's more like a cheerleader, cheering you on with, "You can do it!"

And He's much more than that. He loves you first—before you ever lose a pound. And losing weight won't make Him love you any more. He'll help fill up the hungers you have, heal the brokenness you feel, empower your motivation, and fill you with courage and hope. He'll give you insight into the steps you need to take and celebrate each and every positive aspect of your transformation.

God wants you at your best. He needs you at your best. He values your role in His kingdom, and He'll use you in every way that you let Him. God loves you just the way you are. And He loves you enough to help you become the person He created you to be, weight and all.

A FEW QUESTIONS

Q: Could thyroid problems be causing my weight problem?

A: About one in ten women develop a thyroid disorder at some point, and that makes controlling weight more difficult. If you are hypothyroid, taking thyroid medication can help you lose weight, but you'll still need to make the necessary dietary and exercise changes in order to be successful.

Q: Did menopause cause my weight problem?

A: Many women gain weight around the menopause transition. We know it's not primarily due to hormones because women who take estrogen for menopausal symptoms gain the same amount of weight as women who don't. A woman's metabolism changes around the time of menopause, which means her body burns fuel differently. Many women need to modify their eating habits and exercise pattern in order to prevent gaining weight after menopause.

Chapter 11

CANCER PREVENTION FOR WOMEN

Ask anyone to list the ten words that incite the most fear in their mind, and *cancer* is certain to be one of them. I've seen that fear in a patient's face when I tell them they need a biopsy to rule out cancer. I've felt my own heart beat faster when someone in my family was diagnosed with cancer. Utter the words "It's cancer," and the person you're talking to is not likely to hear much of anything you say after that.

For women, cancer often touches the most intimate parts of who we are. The parts of us that make us women have betrayed us. Breasts, cervix, uterus, ovaries—who am I if I lose those parts of me? We know intellectually that that's not an accurate depiction of our femininity, but the feelings of loss can go very deep.

How much better to forego the experience of cancer altogether. We know a lot of ways to decrease the likelihood of ever having to hear that dreaded six-letter word, and some of this chapter will deal with cancer prevention in general. We'll also talk about ways to decrease your risk for some of the most common cancers affecting women.

"It Won't Happen to Me"

I hope that's true! But statistics say that about one in three of us will develop cancer during our lifetime, and about one in five of us will die from the disease.[1] Simply ignoring the possibility is not smart, especially when the choices you make today can greatly impact which side of those statistics you end up on in the future.

Each of the millions of cells in your body is controlled by thousands of genes contained within the cell nucleus, the control center of the cell. Each gene is a coded message written in the DNA (deoxyribonucleic acid) telling the cell how to behave in a certain way. Some genes code simple messages, such as "blue eyes" or "red hair." Some genes code more complex messages detailing how the cell takes in nutrients, what hormone the cell is to manufacture, how often the cell divides, or even how long the cell survives. Some genes are tumor-suppressor genes, specifically tasked with keeping the cell from "going rogue."

Mistakes called *mutations* may happen in any of these genes. When a mutation is present in an egg or sperm, it is then passed on to every cell in the body as that individual grows. The worst such mutations can lead to genetic illnesses, such as cystic fibrosis or sickle-cell anemia. Other mutations can happen in any given cell at any time during a person's life. DNA is a complex molecule, and there are many reasons breakage or other damage may occur. Most of these mutations are detected and quickly fixed by the cell's very efficient repair system.

Sometimes one of these mutations happens in a vital gene responsible for controlling how the cell divides or repairs itself, or in a tumor-suppressor gene. If that mutation isn't detected and repaired, the abnormal cell may begin to divide quickly without the normal control mechanisms in place. The repair mechanism itself may be incomplete or faulty. Further multiplication may lead some of the abnormal daughter cells to invade other tissues or break free and then grow in other places in the body

> **Health Tip**
>
> *Anything damaging your body's cells and DNA can increase your risk of cancer. Anything protecting your body's cells and DNA and improving their repair mechanisms can decrease your risk of cancer.*

(this is what's called *metastasis*), and the process of cancer continues.

And now you've had a mini-course on cancer!

Most of what we know about cancer fits into this story. Radiation, certain viruses, or certain chemicals, such as those contained in tobacco, can damage DNA directly or interfere with the cell's repair mechanisms. Certain other lifestyle factors can do the same. And other lifestyle practices improve your body's ability to prevent or detect and repair those frequent DNA mutations, thereby preventing cancer from developing at all.

So how does a woman go about protecting her cells' DNA? Let's look at how we can limit exposure to the things that mess up our genes while getting plenty of the things that help keep our body's cells in good repair.

CANCER PREVENTION BASICS

Now that you understand the basic story of how cancer begins, much of what we know about cancer prevention is easy to understand. Anything that damages your body's cells and their DNA is suspect. Anything that helps keep your DNA strong or helps your body detect and repair mistakes quickly is beneficial.

Here are some things you can do to help your body keep every cell's DNA in good working order and limit cancer-causing mutations.

1. Don't smoke—and stay away from secondhand smoke too.

You know this; you've heard it for years. But now you understand more about why. Thirty percent of all cancer deaths are caused by tobacco.[2] There are dozens of cancer-causing chemicals in tobacco and tobacco smoke that damage the DNA in the cells of not only your lungs but also many other organs. Tobacco use leads to a significantly increased risk of cancer in all areas of the respiratory tract (mouth, nose, lips, throat, sinuses) and also the esophagus, stomach, pancreas, kidney, bladder, uterus, cervix, colon, ovary, and one form of leukemia.

Wow! And you thought tobacco only damaged your lungs. Remember, the chemicals in tobacco are also absorbed into your bloodstream and can damage the DNA in cells you never thought could be affected.

This isn't a criticism of you if you use tobacco. It's addictive, and it can be very tough to quit. If you need help to stop using tobacco, check out appendix B for some helpful ideas. Your risk of cancer begins to decrease as soon as you quit.

2. Stay active, and manage your weight.

You know weight and exercise affect a person's risk of heart disease, but you may not realize how important they are for decreasing your risk of cancer. The American Cancer Society reports that up to one-third of all cancer deaths are due to the combination of poor nutrition, lack of exercise, and excess weight.[3] One in three! Being sedentary and being overweight both increase your risk of

> **Health Tip**
>
> *One-third of all cancer deaths are due to the combination of poor nutrition, lack of exercise, and excess weight.*

postmenopausal breast cancer and cancer of the colon, uterus, pancreas, liver, kidney, and others.

Why would body weight or physical activity affect your risk of cancer? Research doesn't give a simple answer. We know, however, that obesity changes your metabolism in many ways, including increasing insulin resistance and increasing estrogen levels. These factors, and perhaps others, may damage a cell's DNA, increasing the risk of mutations and cancer.

Physical exercise not only helps control your weight, but it increases oxygen delivery and blood flow throughout your body, helping your cells be more efficient at detecting and repairing any DNA damage and eliminating any toxins in your bloodstream. Exercise decreases blood levels of insulin and related proteins, and that decreases stress-induced damage to your cell's DNA.

3. Eat healthy.

This is the third part of that triple whammy of poor nutrition, lack of exercise, and obesity that causes one-third of all cancer deaths. The wrong kinds of food dump stress-producing chemicals on your body's cells, increase insulin levels, and add to your waistline—all bad for your cells' DNA. The "bad stuff" includes processed and red meat, refined grain products, and sweetened beverages.

Eating healthy provides your body's cells with the ideal mechanisms to protect and repair DNA. Research repeatedly documents the cancer-preventing value of a diet rich in fruits and vegetables, whole grains, and fish or poultry while limiting processed foods and red meat. Cruciferous vegetables, such as broccoli, brussels sprouts, kale, and cauliflower, are particularly strong at preventing cancer.

Antioxidants are phytonutrients found in fruits and vegetables, and many individual molecules in this group have been studied for their cancer-fighting properties. No single antioxidant, when used alone, has been consistently proven to prevent cancer, perhaps because the phytonutrients in fruits and veggies work best when they're together in the combinations God built into our food plants.

4. Limit environmental exposures.

This one gets most of the press coverage, but all exposures taken together (occupational exposure and environmental pollutants, both natural and man-made) account for only about 6 percent of all cancer deaths.[4] That doesn't mean we should be complacent. Asbestos, hydrocarbons, various solvents and dyes, and chemicals used by leatherworkers are some of the best-established cancer-causing chemicals. Smog, cell phones, pesticides, formaldehyde in building materials—the best research indicates all these have, at best, a minimal effect on your risk of cancer.

We know too much radiation causes cancer; that's why you wear a lead apron while getting dental X-rays. Naturally occurring radiation in the form of radon is more common than many people realize. It's a good idea to test the radon level in your home; inexpensive kits are available at many hardware stores. If the level is more than 4 picocuries per liter (pCu/L), take steps to fix the problem.

5. Don't worship the sun.

Tanning beds, sunbathing, and other normal outdoor summer activities will increase your risk for skin cancers, including the deadly melanoma. Ultraviolet rays damage your skin cells' DNA, and the healing process that happens after a sunburn may damage it even more. Your risk is higher if, like me, you have fair skin. Sunscreen can decrease your risk, but that brings up the question of using more chemicals. A hat and light, loose-fitting clothing that covers your body are at least as effective. If you're going to be outside, do something to protect yourself. If you'd ever known someone with melanoma, you wouldn't worry as much about the comparatively insignificant chemicals in sunscreen.

6. Beware of viruses.

Most viruses don't cause cancer, but a few can induce infected cells to become malignant by altering their DNA. The human papillomavirus (HPV) is spread by touch. While most varieties of HPV are harmless, at least a dozen strains can cause cancer and are often spread by close contact during either genital or oral sex.

Cervical cancer is a sexually transmitted disease. Almost all cases of cervical cancer are directly caused by HPV, as are many cancers of the anus, vagina, mouth, and throat. The combination of HPV exposure and smoking is especially damaging, since each insult adds damage to the cells' DNA.

HPV usually causes no symptoms early, so the best detection mechanism is having a Pap test that includes HPV testing. (This is covered further in chapter 15.) Vaccines, including Gardasil and Cervarix, are excellent though not perfect protection. The best prevention is a mutually monogamous, lifelong relationship with one husband, which brings your risk to zero.

The hepatitis B and C viruses may cause chronic liver disease and eventually liver cancer. These viruses are only acquired through bodily fluids, such as during sexual contact or from using infected needles. Modern testing of the blood supply makes the risk of hepatitis from a blood transfusion very rare (about 1 in 200,000 to 1 in 2 million). If you develop hepatitis, treatment will significantly decrease the risk of chronic infection, liver damage, and liver cancer.

HIV (human immunodeficiency virus) is still a big scare for some people. The basic facts are still the same: it's only transmitted through bodily fluids. Various forms of cancer are more common in people living with HIV because their body's immune system is less able to fight viruses, such as HPV and hepatitis, or to detect and destroy newly formed precancerous cells containing damaged DNA.

Health Tip

To decrease your risk of cancer by about two-thirds:

- *Don't smoke.*
- *Exercise regularly.*
- *Eat a healthy diet.*
- *Maintain a healthy weight.*
- *Only engage in a mutually monogamous sexual relationship.*
- *Protect your skin from the sun.*

There are a few much-less-common viruses also associated with an increased risk of cancer, but the ones listed here are those you need to know about to make appropriate lifestyle choices.

The bottom line is that if you exercise regularly, eat a healthy diet, are not overweight, and don't smoke, you've just eliminated the causes of 65 percent of cancers. And if you protect your skin from the sun and remain in a lifelong, mutually monogamous relationship, you've eliminated another significant portion of your cancer risk.

Living a perfectly healthy lifestyle doesn't guarantee you won't get cancer, but it gives your body a much better chance of keeping the DNA of your body's cells in good working order. Cancer will be much less likely, and you'll be in a much stronger position to fight cancer if it does happen to you.

GENETICS AND CANCER

Some mutations in our genetic makeup can be inherited from our parents. We know of about fifty hereditary cancer syndromes caused by mutations in specific genes. Approximately 5 to 10 percent of all cancers are related to one of these genetic abnormalities. The genes affected are thought to be those concerned with cell growth or the repair of damaged DNA.

Certain features in a person's individual or family medical history increase the likelihood of one of these hereditary cancer syndromes, including when cancer develops at an unusually early age, when several cancers develop in one individual, when several family members develop the same or similar cancer, or when cancer presents in an unusual way. Perhaps the best known of these conditions is mutations in the BRCA1 and BRCA2 genes, which are associated with breast and ovarian cancer.

Testing for these genetic conditions can be quite complex, and you should think carefully before doing so. Testing usually involves taking your blood along with that of any family members who may also be affected. A genetics counselor is the best person to discuss with you what the test will tell you and what it won't, and to help you think through the decisions involved. No test can tell you whether or not you'll get cancer, but you'll know more about your risks for certain cancers if you decide to be tested. You'll also need to think about how to talk to your family, including children; how to handle privacy issues; and whether you would do anything differently once you knew the results.

One thing is for sure: even if you have a genetic predisposition to a certain type of cancer, following a healthy lifestyle will give your body the best possible chance of fighting any cancer before it starts and dealing with it effectively if it does develop.

BREAST CANCER

If there's anything scarier than the word *cancer* to a woman, it's *breast cancer*. It can happen at any age but most commonly happens after menopause. Several high-profile women who experienced breast cancer have made this one of the better known and better studied forms of cancer.

Many women who develop breast cancer have no risk factors, and others with risk factors never develop breast cancer. But here are some things we know increase a woman's risk: drinking alcohol (more than one drink per day), being overweight, not having a child by age thirty, and (possibly) long-term use of oral contraceptives. Regular physical exercise and breastfeeding decrease a woman's risk somewhat.

Whether or not postmenopausal hormone therapy raises a woman's risk for breast cancer has proved controversial. Dozens of research studies have been done, some of them very large, and not all of them come to the same conclusions. The evidence is moderately strong that using synthetic estrogens and synthetic progestins (such as those contained in Prempro) for more than five years modestly increases a woman's risk for breast cancer. Using estrogen alone hasn't been associated with the same risks; in the large Women's Health Initiative study, use of estrogen alone slightly decreased the risk of breast cancer.[5]

No data exists that directly compares the risk of breast cancer after using synthetic estrogens versus natural estradiol. Specifically, we have no data to indicate the popular compounded bioidentical hormones are safer in this regard. (See more on this in chapter 8.) My own evaluation of the data is that if women using natural estradiol to treat menopausal symptoms have an increased risk of breast cancer, it's very small. Use it only as long as you need it to control your symptoms, and get regular breast checkups. If you don't need progestin, don't use it. If you have a uterus, use natural progesterone to prevent overgrowth of the uterine lining. That's the message I give all my patients, and I think it's the best way to look at all the evidence.

I recommend my patients get mammograms, and there's a whole section about how often, when, and why you should in chapter 15.

CERVICAL CANCER

No HPV, no cervical cancer. It's just that simple. Especially in young women under age thirty, the body's own immune system will get rid of the HPV most of the time. The pathway from HPV infection to cervical cancer is almost always a very slow one. Having regular Pap tests and HPV testing when needed can almost always detect cellular changes long before they become actual cancer. Treatment at that point decreases the risk of cancer developing by about 98 percent.

The availability of Gardasil and Cervarix to vaccinate girls and young women ages nine to twenty-five against HPV has raised a lot of controversy. The vaccines are very effective, though not perfect.

As a gynecologist I know that most young women will have several sexual partners and therefore be exposed to HPV. From that perspective, getting vaccinated is just common sense. Most men infected with HPV have no symptoms and may not be aware they are passing on a potentially deadly virus. This past month alone I've cared for two women dying of cervical cancer who wouldn't be dying if they had been vaccinated against HPV.

Vaccination isn't the only way to prevent cervical cancer. Many Christian parents and adults advocate abstinence-only sex education, and abstinence is certainly the safest way to go. I can't support mandatory HPV vaccination. Because HPV and cervical cancer are sexually transmitted diseases, I don't believe we should force girls to become vaccinated against a threat they can voluntarily choose not to become exposed to. However, no parent can fully predict what their daughter will do in the future. This is a matter parents need to prayerfully consider and talk about openly with their daughters in coming to a thoughtful decision.

UTERINE CANCER

The most common uterine cancer is endometrial cancer, or cancer of the lining of the uterus. Estrogen stimulates the endometrium to grow, and if that process continues unrestricted, cancer will eventually develop. Women who have regular ovulatory menstrual periods have a very low chance of contracting endometrial cancer. The progesterone produced by the ovaries after ovulation stops the growth of the endometrium, and the tissue then sloughs off during menses.

Women who don't ovulate regularly don't have that regular progesterone protection and are at higher risk. Women who are overweight have more estrogen in their body and are also less likely to ovulate regularly, thereby significantly increasing their risk for endometrial cancer.

After menopause, the risk for endometrial cancer increases in part because there is no longer any progesterone being produced to protect the endometrium. The amounts of estrogen most women's ovaries make after menopause is not high enough to stimulate the endometrium, but the estrogen produced by the extra fatty tissue in women who are overweight makes this a significant problem. This is also why women who are prescribed estrogen after menopause need to take some form of progesterone unless they've had a hysterectomy.

Any vaginal bleeding after menopause is cause for concern and should lead to an ultrasound and/or biopsy of the endometrium. The only exception would be a woman using hormonal therapy in a way that vaginal bleeding is expected; a biopsy might then be unnecessary.

OVARIAN CANCER

The absence of early warning signs makes ovarian cancer one of the toughest cancers to detect early and to effectively treat. Besides smoking and obesity, the one risk factor you need to know about is talc. Some women use powder (such as baby powder) in the genital area to feel fresh and dry. Small bits of talc may be drawn into the vagina, into the uterus, and through the fallopian tubes, increasing the risk of ovarian cancer. If you wish to use something to feel fresh and dry, use cornstarch. Stay away from talc.

You can do other things, too, that lower your risk of ovarian cancer. Having babies significantly lowers your risk, as does using oral contraceptives (or any contraceptive that prevents ovulation). That protection lasts for several years after you stop using contraception. There is also a potential benefit of removing a woman's fallopian tubes, as recent evidence indicates ovarian cancer may often begin in the fallopian tubes. If you need a hysterectomy, ask your doctor about leaving your ovaries in place but removing your tubes.

LUNG CANCER

You may wonder why lung cancer is a topic in a book devoted to women's health. The sad news is that more women die from lung cancer than from any other cancer—more than breast cancer, ovarian cancer, cervical cancer, or uterine cancer. That's a surprise to many people, but it's true.

And I think you know the reason why. It's not that every case of lung cancer is caused by smoking, but the majority of cases are. If you need some help quitting, please get it! And check out appendix B for more on this topic.

COLORECTAL CANCER

Eating a diet rich in high-fat animal products, being overweight, smoking, and being inactive all increase your risk of colorectal cancer.

This is an equal-opportunity destroyer, affecting almost as many women as men.

It's also a disease from which nobody should have to die. Early detection can be very effective, and there are many options. We'll cover this more in chapter 15.

DON'T GIVE UP HOPE

I hate cancer too. It's ugly, insidious, and greedy. It's caused far too many families to miss out on the many years their wives, daughters, and mothers should have been there.

If you've read this chapter and see a number of things in your lifestyle that increase your risk of cancer, don't give up. Your chance of cancer begins to decrease the moment you make a positive change.

So, how about it? Make the decision to stop smoking. Start walking every evening. Change out some processed food for fruits and veggies. The DNA in all your body's cells will thank you.

A FEW QUESTIONS

Q: What if I've already had cancer? Is there anything I can do to prevent it from coming back?

A: Yes! While there are no guarantees, following the lifestyle tips in this chapter will do a lot to keep your immune system strong. Refraining from smoking, eating a diet rich in fruits and vegetables, and managing your weight and your stress will give your body the best opportunity to fight any remaining or new cancer cells that develop. For example, research demonstrates that people who already have lung cancer live longer if they quit smoking even after their diagnosis.[6] Of course, it's important to follow your doctor's advice regarding follow-up and treatment.

Q: Are there any supplements that will help prevent cancer?

A: There are no long-term, good-quality research studies proving that any supplement prevents cancer, for now. However, phytonutrient supplements have been proven to prevent DNA damage, which may well lessen the risk of many cancers.[7] This is another reason why I recommend Juice Plus+, known as "fruits and vegetables in a capsule." (See chapter 17 for more on this option.)

Chapter 12
DISEASES OLDER WOMEN FACE

WHEN YOU'RE NINETEEN, you can't imagine ever being anything but strong and healthy. You take outrageous chances and believe the worst will never happen to you. You're invincible.

When you're thirty-nine, you wish you could stop the clock. If you didn't stop counting birthdays at twenty-nine, you certainly do now. You're likely either an overstressed mama or worried about the ticking of your biological clock.

When you're fifty-nine, you know you should have listened to all those health messages years ago. You're feeling the results of decades of habits, either good or bad. If only you could have a serious talk with your nineteen-year-old self!

In most years prior to about 1920, more people died of influenza than died of heart disease. Tuberculosis was the second-leading cause of death, and cancer and stroke were far down the list. Since 1930, heart disease has been number one and cancer number two. In just the last few years, Alzheimer's disease, diabetes, and chronic respiratory illnesses, such as COPD (chronic obstructive pulmonary disease), have appeared among the leading causes of death.[1]

What does this say about our lifestyle? We've gotten much better at treating most infectious diseases, but lifestyle illnesses are wreaking more and more havoc among us. Rates of heart disease and stroke have decreased somewhat as more doctors and patients take high blood pressure seriously, but the increase in some of these other illnesses is very concerning.

This side of heaven, we each must die of something. But let's make the years we have left the best years possible. There's no need to be any sicker than absolutely necessary. There's no need to have one unnecessary day of pain or disability or miss out on one day of adventure or love that we don't have to. There's no need to leave this earth one day before our work is done.

Let's get down to business doing what we can to stamp out disease and to live long and healthy lives. Let's talk about some common diseases older women face and hit them right in the mouth.

HEART DISEASE

You may be aware of the Go Red for Women campaign by the American Heart Association,[2] devoted to raising awareness that one in three American women die of heart disease and stroke. The campaign helps women find ways to avoid being another statistic. And the numbers are scary: if they have a heart attack, women are more likely than men to die as a result, and they're more likely to have a second heart attack. As a group, we are most afraid of breast cancer, but heart disease kills many more of us.

Many women may not be as concerned about this problem because prior to menopause, women have a lower rate of heart disease than men do. Most scientists believe that ovarian hormones, especially estrogen, offer significant protection to a woman's heart and blood vessels during her reproductive years. Once those hormones decrease after menopause, that protection is gone, and women quickly catch up to men in the heart disease arena.

Health Tip
Following a healthy lifestyle over time can decrease your risk of heart disease to only 8 percent of what it otherwise would have been. That's a 92 percent decrease.

But it doesn't have to be that way. A recent study showed that women who followed a healthy lifestyle during their younger years decreased their risk of developing heart disease during middle age by 92 percent.[3] The lifestyle factors that showed up as important were not smoking, physical activity at least two-and-a-half hours per week, less than seven hours of television viewing per week, a normal body mass index, a healthy diet (in the top 40 percent of the measured criteria), and not drinking more than one alcoholic drink each day. This study followed young women beginning in their twenties. If you're already living that healthy lifestyle, you can rest assured you probably won't get heart disease.

But what if you're not living that healthy right now? What if you're forty and overweight, or fifty and your only exercise is the few steps you take from your car to your office and back? And only one hour of television a day—really? That could make many of us want to give up.

I wish the researchers had measured time spent sitting rather than time spent watching television. Perhaps TV viewing was easier to measure. The real issue probably isn't the number of hours the silver screen is turned on but the amount of time spent sitting on your backside. A strong and growing body of research has linked the number of hours a person spends sitting each day to death from all kinds of causes, regardless of whether they engage in physical activity at other times or not. Sitting can kill you.

This really shouldn't surprise you. You've probably heard about these health habits many times. What's impressive is how dramatic the difference is between those who adopt a healthy lifestyle and those who don't. Said another way, for every one hundred women who die of heart disease and have an unhealthy lifestyle, only eight women who consistently follow those six healthy lifestyle practices will die of heart disease. That's 92 percent less!

The important thing to notice is that these behaviors are all things you can control. Changing your lifestyle may be difficult, but it *is* within your power to do. Don't be fooled into thinking it's too late for you or that the necessary changes are too big. Any small action you take today will add up to positive results in the future.

Both diabetes and abnormal blood lipids increase your chances for developing heart disease. Blood lipids include "good" cholesterol (high-density lipoproteins, or HDL), "bad" cholesterol (low-density lipoproteins, or LDL), and triglycerides. You can only know about these conditions by taking the appropriate blood tests. Even if your levels are abnormal, following a healthy diet and getting adequate exercise may dramatically improve these conditions. If that's not enough, treating them with medication will significantly decrease your risk of heart disease.

If you need to make some lifestyle changes, here are three critical steps you must take:

1. **Decide on your why.** Simply saying "I don't want to get heart disease" won't be a big enough reason to motivate you to stick with any changes you need to make. Instead, take the time to think through a reason that grabs at your emotions and your will. Perhaps you want to stay healthy long enough to see your grandchildren grow up. Perhaps you want to feel vibrant and strong, physically and mentally. Perhaps you want to have the energy to accomplish what you see as God's purpose for you. Make it specific. Write it down.

2. **Start slow.** We all know how long a crash diet or
   a sudden intense workout program is likely to last.
   It's not! Choose one lifestyle factor, and make one
   change this week in a positive direction. Take a
   twenty-minute walk after dinner with your husband
   or a friend. Make an appointment to talk with your
   doctor about stopping smoking. Substitute something
   healthier for one processed food this week. Then next
   week, make another small but sustainable change.
   Keep doing this each week until 80 to 90 percent of
   your lifestyle is healthy. These little changes add up.

3. **Celebrate success.** How much you weigh next week
   isn't nearly as important as how much you will weigh
   five years from now. It's the same with your eating patterns and your physical activity. Celebrate the healthy
   changes you're actually making more than the results
   you have less control over. Remember, you can control what you eat and how often you get up and walk
   around instead of sitting. Tell your friends. Post your
   success on Facebook. Do something nice for yourself.
   Rejoice in the positive direction you're choosing to
   take your life.

Most of all, remember it's never too late. Eating more healthfully,
being more physically active, and not smoking will all decrease your
blood pressure, improve your cholesterol level, and make your heart and
blood vessels healthier, whether or not you lose any extra weight. And
shedding some excess pounds magnifies those benefits even further.

Even after a woman has developed heart disease, has had a heart
attack, or has had bypass surgery, these positive lifestyle changes will
improve her heart health and decrease her chances for further heart
problems. What you do today *will* make a difference in your tomorrow.

DIABETES

During the last fifty years, the rates of diabetes have increased steadily,
and most rapidly in the last twenty years.[4] Complications of diabetes—
heart disease, loss of eyesight, kidney failure, and lower extremity ampu-
tations—are increasing too. Since 1980 the number of individuals with

diabetes has more than tripled. Today twenty-one million Americans know they have diabetes, and the Centers for Disease Control estimates another eight million have diabetes but don't yet know it. Diabetes is one of the most rapidly increasing leading causes of death.

The increase in type 2 diabetes is directly linked to the increase in obesity in our culture. A graph showing the increase in diabetes can be almost superimposed on a graph showing the increase in obesity. Furthermore, the states with the largest percentage of obese adults also have the highest rates of diabetes. Genetics and factors in our environment do play a role, but diabetes is one of the clearest consequences of all the extra pounds we're carrying around.

How does diabetes happen? Your body's cells—especially your brain cells—need glucose to function, and your digestive system breaks down the carbohydrates you eat into glucose and other sugars. Once it's absorbed into your bloodstream, insulin shuttles glucose into your body's cells, where it's either used for energy or stored. When the body's cells can't respond efficiently to insulin or when the pancreas (where insulin is made) isn't able to keep up with the demand, glucose increases in the blood. That's diabetes. The chronic increase in blood sugar damages blood vessels, especially in the heart, eyes, and kidneys, hence all the complications of diabetes.

When high levels of both insulin and blood sugar are present in your blood, your body's cells can quickly become resistant to insulin. Your cells can develop selective hearing, just like you can. If the radio is on at your workplace or if a coworker constantly complains out loud, you learn to tune out those sounds. Soon you don't even hear them. In the same way, insulin resistance is your body's cells tuning out insulin.

Health Tip

Losing 5 to 7 percent of your body weight can cut your risk of diabetes by one-third. If you weigh three hundred pounds, that means losing just fifteen pounds.

Insulin resistance increases with increased body weight. At first your cells can keep up with the extra demand. Your blood sugar may increase only slightly. At this point, you have prediabetes—along with at least eighty-six million other Americans. If that relatively mild insulin resistance continues, both your pancreas and your cells' ability to respond to insulin will wear out, and you'll develop full diabetes. That explanation is a little simplistic, but it explains much of what we know about this disease.

The good news? It doesn't take much to turn around your risk for diabetes. If you're obese (as one-third of Americans are), losing 5 to 7 percent of your body weight can cut your risk of diabetes by one-third. In other words, if you weigh two hundred pounds, losing just ten pounds may be enough to keep you from becoming another statistic. If you already have diabetes, losing a modest amount of weight will decrease your need for medication and may eliminate the need altogether. And if losing the first ten pounds can make that much difference, think how much losing more can do.

Simple exercise, such as walking, cycling, or swimming, is an effective way to lower blood sugar. When you move your muscles, they gobble up glucose like blood-sugar-burning machines. All your body's cells become more sensitive to insulin, and the vicious cycle is reversed. The effect of thirty minutes of walking continues for hours after you're done and begins to improve your metabolism long before you shed any pounds. As you lose weight, the effect becomes even greater.

What you eat certainly plays a role. Limiting calories is important, but it's at least as important to limit processed foods. Simple carbohydrates like sugar and refined grains are quickly absorbed and raise blood sugar and insulin levels rapidly. It has the effect of shouting at your body's cells; they'll soon learn to tune out those signals. Complex carbohydrates like vegetables and whole grains are absorbed much more slowly. Think of this like whispering to your body's cells; they'll have to listen up and pay attention to get the glucose they need—and that's a very good thing for preventing, controlling, or reversing diabetes.

If you have a strong family history of diabetes, you may have to work harder than others to keep your blood-sugar system healthy. While no one can guarantee you'll never develop diabetes, you can dramatically lessen your risks if you exercise regularly, maintain a healthy weight, and eat a diet based largely on healthy protein, fruits and vegetables, and whole grains.

Diabetes is not inevitable. It's one of those lifestyle diseases that you can kick right in the mouth.

OSTEOPOROSIS

It's easy to think of bones as the wooden frame inside a chair: solid, stable, and only breakable with a large amount of force. But in reality, our bones are constantly changing. They are living things.

Each bone has its vital blood supply that provides the oxygen and nutrients the bone needs to remain alive. Our bones respond to hormones, stress, diet, and things in our environment. They're worth taking care of.

You know calcium is important for bone health, but that's only part of the story. If your bones were made of solid mineral, they'd be so heavy you couldn't move your limbs. You know that larger bones have hollow spaces within them containing marrow. But even the so-called solid portions of bone aren't really solid. All bone is actually a matrix of material structured similar to a sponge. Such a matrix allows bones to withstand a lot more mechanical stress than their size alone might indicate.

Some bone cells, called osteoclasts, are constantly removing bits of old bone to make room for new. Other bone cells, called osteoblasts, are constantly laying down bits of new bone. The thickness and strength of the bone matrix is determined by the balance between these two processes, and osteoporosis develops when the creation of new bone doesn't keep up with removal of old bone. The matrix becomes brittle, and simple forces, such as bending over, a cough, or a mild fall, can lead to fractures.

Such osteoporosis-related fractures cause a lot of disability. Vertebral fractures in the back cause pain—sometimes debilitating—and loss of height and mobility. Hip fractures may result in surgery, prolonged nursing home stays, or permanent loss of mobility. Women who fracture a hip have up to a five-times-higher risk of dying within a year than women who don't, in part because of surgical complications or blood clots due to prolonged immobility. Osteoporosis is an expensive and painful problem.

We normally reach our peak bone mass in our twenties. That's the time at which our bone matrix is the strongest and densest. You'll never be able to get more bone than you have at that time. That's why it's important for girls and young women to engage in lifestyle behaviors that help their bone density develop to its maximum: regular exercise, adequate

Health Tip

To maintain healthy bones:

- *Exercise regularly.*
- *Eat protein at most meals.*
- *Get at least 1,000 mg of calcium daily, ideally from your diet.*
- *Consider vitamin D blood testing, and take extra only if needed.*

calcium intake, and a healthy diet. Eating disorders and intense sports programs such as gymnastics or dance that delay a girl's menstrual periods and focus on extreme thinness may significantly lower a young woman's peak bone mass and increase her risk for osteoporosis later. So does excessive alcohol use while young.

Peak bone mass is like a bank account: the larger the initial deposit, the longer you can make withdrawals without going broke (no pun intended). From the time of peak bone mass, each one of us begins to lose a tiny bit of bone every year. Between about age twenty and age fifty, that bone loss is very slow, but it speeds up significantly with the loss of estrogen at menopause. Having more bone mass to start with means you can lose a lot more before your bones become thin or brittle enough to risk fractures.

As with many diseases, genetics makes a difference. Asian and Caucasian women have a greater risk for osteoporosis, as their peak bone mass is less than women of other ethnic backgrounds. The rate of bone loss is also somewhat genetically determined. If your mother or grandmother developed a "dowager's hump" or lost height as she grew older, she probably had osteoporosis, and that increases your risk as well.

Health Tip

Peak bone mass is like a bank account: the larger the initial deposit, the longer you can make withdrawals without going broke. Your largest deposits of bone mass happen by age twenty.

Osteoporosis is one area where being overweight does not increase your risks. Extra body weight puts extra stress on bones, and that can make them stronger. Being underweight for any reason increases your risk significantly.

You can do a lot to slow down bone loss and preserve the bones you have for as long as possible. Those cells that lay down new bone respond to stress. The good kind of stress, that is—mechanical stress. That means it's good to engage in weight-bearing exercises, such as walking, jogging, running, dancing, skiing, or weight training. Sports where you're running or jumping are good for you too. Non-weight-bearing exercise, such as swimming, cycling, or using a machine such as an elliptical, are great for your heart but don't add significant strength to your bones. Strength training is also helpful, as it increases the tension your muscles place on your bones, which is what they need.

What you eat is also important. The link between protein intake and bone health has been a little controversial. More animal protein in the diet has been blamed for loss of bone mineral, but that hasn't turned out to be as big a factor as many believed. Not getting enough protein in the diet can definitely lead to loss of bone tissue, though that's only likely to be a major problem for women older than sixty-five. The consensus? We probably need more protein than is generally recommended to keep our bones at their best. That doesn't mean buying protein powders. It does mean you should try to eat protein—eggs, milk, lean fish or poultry, legumes, and the like—at most meals.

You need 1,000 mg per day of calcium prior to age fifty and 1,200 mg per day after that. It's best to get that from your diet through milk and milk products, green leafy vegetables, soy products, calcium-fortified cereals, orange juice, and the like. Taking extra calcium as supplements has been associated with kidney stones and heart problems, so focus first on making sure calcium is present in your diet. If you're older and don't use a lot of milk products, you probably need a calcium tablet each day.

Vitamin D is one of the most talked about and controversial topics in nutritional science today. We know for certain that this "sunshine vitamin" is critically important for bone health, but there's a lot of debate over how much is necessary. And the debate is even louder when it comes to how much vitamin D affects a whole host of other health issues. If you spend time outdoors, you're probably just fine. If you use sunscreen daily and are rarely in the sun, or if you're over age seventy, you probably need 600–800 IU (international units) a day. (See chapter 15 for more about vitamin D blood testing.)

And then there's the acid/alkaline issue. Acidic foods, such as sodas or meat, can potentially leach some calcium out of your bones. More than one soda a day provides too much phosphoric acid for your body to buffer safely, and your body will take calcium out of your bones to make up the difference—one more reason to cut sodas from your diet! Fruits and vegetables provide the ideal alkaline alternative to any acid-producing foods you eat, such as protein. Focus on increasing how much fresh produce you eat rather than trying to measure or limit protein in your diet.

If you already have osteoporosis, you can limit the chance of any (or more) fractures occurring. Make sure you're getting enough calcium and vitamin D in your diet or through supplements. Unless your doctor has told you not to do so, walking regularly and engaging in strength training and balance exercises will improve your mobility and decrease your risk of falls. Take steps to decrease the chance for falls at home, such as removing throw rugs and ensuring stairs or other risky areas are well lit.

Medications including estrogen, bisphosphonates, and others are useful for stabilizing bone loss and decreasing fracture risk in women with established osteoporosis. If you choose to use estrogen to treat menopausal symptoms, it will help maintain your bone density and decrease your chances for osteoporosis. Bisphosphonates can be challenging medications to take, and how long to take them is controversial. If you take them, follow your doctor's instructions carefully.

And long live your bones!

You Can Make a Difference

We've talked about heart disease, cancer, diabetes, and osteoporosis. All of these diseases are lifestyle related, which means you can do a lot to prevent them. I see women every day who just feel bad, and that may be the most important "disease" of all. I can promise you that if you exercise regularly and reduce processed foods in your diet, that disease may well be cured.

But there's more we need to say about aging. Are those "senior moments" really Alzheimer's disease? You can do a lot to stay younger longer. Let's turn to that discussion next.

A Few Questions

Q: How can I find out my risk of having a heart attack?

A: If you already have a diagnosis of heart disease or diabetes, you're at high risk and should talk with your doctor about this question. If you're twenty or older, there's a helpful online free tool based on the Framingham Heart Study that you can use to estimate your risk of having a heart attack in the coming ten years. You can use this information to talk with your doctor, and to make lifestyle changes to decrease your risk if necessary. You can find it here: http://cvdrisk .nhlbi.nih.gov/.

Q: How can I find out my risk of having an osteoporosis-related fracture?

A: The FRAX tool is a software program developed in conjunction with the World Health Organization designed to provide middle-aged and older individuals with their probability of having an osteoporosis-related fracture during the coming ten years. You can use this free tool online yourself at www.shef.ac.uk/FRAX. Click on the Calculation Tool tab at the top, choose the region of the world where you live, and enter your information. If your risk is high, be sure to discuss this information with your doctor.

Chapter 13
STAYING YOUNGER LONGER

YOUR FACE AT twenty is the result of your parents' choices. Your face at eighty is the result of your own choices. Wrinkles or no wrinkles; that's a sobering thought—and I'm not even talking about the more than $260 billion being spent every year on antiaging products and services.[1]

What is it that we fear about getting older? Loss of physical beauty? Loss of physical health? Loss of independence? Loss of mental capacity? Loss of time to accomplish or experience all we desire? All those fears look at aging as a series of losses. And perhaps in some ways that's true. Just knowing the world will one day go on without us is a rather unpleasant thought.

The American poet Dylan Thomas expressed it this way:

> Do not go gentle into that good night,
> Old age should burn and rave at close of day;
> Rage, rage against the dying of the light.[2]

Growing older has always been a challenge. Moses wrote, "Our days may come to seventy years, or eighty, if our strength endures; yet the best of them are but trouble and sorrow, for they quickly pass, and we fly away" (Ps. 90:10).

I believe our raging against the finiteness of our existence is evidence that we were made for eternity. In our innermost being we sense that God didn't create us for seventy or eighty or even one hundred years. Death is an imposter, and growing old is hard!

But we can still grow old gracefully, even as we do so under protest. Whatever your reasons for raging against getting old, poor health is not inevitable. You and I have things to do, people to see, and places to go. We have a mission on this earth to accomplish, and we need to stick around for as long and with as much vitality as we can.

You really can stay younger longer.

Attitudes About Aging

In the past two decades a remarkable body of research has demonstrated that attitudes about aging are important for one's health as one gets older. Those who value and respect the wisdom and maturity that aging can provide remain happier, healthier, and active much longer. Those who approach aging with anxiety and fear are more likely to develop sickness and disability. And those who generally view aging in a positive light are able to recover from even severe disability more readily.[3]

I don't know about you, but I wouldn't want to be twenty again, at least not without knowing what I know now. There are many benefits of maturity that we would do well to remember. If you've paid attention to your life, you've received a priceless education that has little or nothing to do with academic schooling or degrees. Simply noticing things about your life and about the world, reflecting on them, and adjusting your behavior accordingly can be a rich source of wisdom.

Here are a few of the things you might have learned:

+ Worrying too much about what other people think isn't useful. You can't please everyone all the time.
+ Some risks are worth taking, even if you're afraid. The best things rarely happen to those who always play it safe.
+ People are more important than money or things. Investing in relationships creates more value than anything else you can do.
+ Small things are important. Daily habits add up to big results, whether in physical health, the financial arena, personal relationships, or spiritual growth.
+ This life won't go on forever. The legacy you leave behind is all that will remain here after you're gone.

Have you ever wished you could have a talk with your younger self? Well, have a talk with the self you are now, whatever your age. Extract all the value you can from your experiences up to this point in life, and determine to make the years you have left the best years of your life.

ALZHEIMER'S DISEASE

You probably either know or know of someone who has developed dementia as they got older, Alzheimer's disease being the most common form. Trouble with short-term memory is often the first symptom, followed by symptoms such as difficulty with judgment, confusion, difficulty performing familiar tasks, personality changes, and loss of long-term memory.

"Senior moments" may lead many middle-aged women to worry if these are early signs of dementia. Forgetting where you left your keys or missing an appointment because you forgot can be scary. It's reassuring to know that most people experience such "senior moments" as they get older, and only rarely do these indicate impending dementia. There is no need to worry unless these moments are accompanied by other symptoms such as those listed above or they begin to affect your daily functioning. Other people who know you well can also provide feedback; if your spouse notices a personality change or if your coworkers are concerned you're no longer doing your job adequately, it's time for further evaluation.

Alzheimer's disease is a complex disorder involving the death of brain cells. Tangles involving the neurons in the brain, deposits of abnormal proteins such as amyloid, and other specific changes all contribute to this cell death. As more brain cells die, the remaining brain cells eventually become unable to pick up important functions such as memory, communication, and judgment.

Dr. Carol Says...

"If you want to remain mentally alert as you age, care for your brain as you care for your heart: exercise regularly, eat a healthy diet, and don't smoke."

Genetics plays a role in some cases of Alzheimer's disease. Only 5 percent of Alzheimer's is so-called early onset (happening before age sixty) and associated with one of three known genetic defects. In most cases, your genetic heritage may affect the vulnerability of your brain cells to various lifestyle or environmental insults, but usually there is much you can do to delay or perhaps prevent the loss of brain function that happens with dementia.

Not all dementia is Alzheimer's disease. Other common causes include medication side effects; chronic alcoholism; progressive small blockages in the blood vessels in the brain; or certain thyroid, kidney,

or liver disorders. Severe emotional distress, such as post-traumatic
stress disorder or complicated grief after the loss of a loved one, can
also mimic many of the symptoms of dementia.

Dementia including Alzheimer's disease is becoming one of the
most expensive health problems in our culture. Alzheimer's disease is
currently the sixth leading cause of death in America, but the financial and personal costs are much higher. The National Institutes of
Health reports that direct costs for health care and personal care for
those with dementia total up to $215 billion each year, greater than
the costs for heart disease or cancer.[4] If one adds the value of unpaid
caregiving by family and friends, the true costs are probably double
that amount.

All these factors should appropriately make you, me, and society
interested in doing all we can to prevent dementia. Research is not
definitive in many of these areas, but the evidence is quite convincing.
Here are things you can do to keep your brain healthier longer:

- **Eat a healthy diet, exercise regularly, and don't smoke.**
  What's good for your heart is also good for your brain.
  Vegetables, fruits, and regular exercise protect the blood vessels in your brain and give your brain cells the ammunition
  they need to withstand insults from either the environment
  around you or your genetic background.

- **Control your weight.** Among all the other health risks of
  obesity, people who are overweight develop Alzheimer's disease more frequently than those who are not. Improving your
  entire metabolism with weight loss is very good for your
  brain cells.

- **Control high blood pressure and diabetes.** These health
  problems seriously increase one's risk for dementia. And here
  we go again with that familiar refrain: eat healthy, exercise,
  lose weight, and take medication when indicated.

- **Remain socially and mentally active.** Reading, playing music,
  learning new things, or conducting other mental exercise helps
  keep your brain healthier longer. So does nurturing close personal relationships, such as a healthy marriage or being part of
  a close group of friends or church group.

+ **Deal with anxiety and depression.** People with psychological distress have a higher chance of developing dementia.[5]
Ouch! That may be because such distress makes your brain
more vulnerable to other damaging factors. Managing stress
well and perhaps using medication when needed will help
your brain stay healthy.

+ **Pursue your life's purpose.** Fascinating research shows
that those who believe their life has a purpose and are intent
on accomplishing that purpose remain mentally alert and
productive much longer, with a lower risk of developing
Alzheimer's disease.[6] God put you here for a reason!

Dementia is not inevitable. You can't guarantee how well your
mind will function in the future, but there is much you can do to hit
dementia right in the mouth.

PRESERVE YOUR SKIN

Oh, how vain we are! Chances are fairly good you've contributed your
share to the $260 billion yearly sales of antiaging products and ser-
vices. Whether it's buying into antiaging creams, injections of botox or
dermal fillers, or cosmetic surgery, we do a lot to look younger.

By the way, why is that? What's wrong with a mature look?

Truthfully, as a senior woman, I understand the desire to have full,
healthy-looking hair; clear, bright eyes; and smooth, even, youthful-
looking skin. Stressing over every gray hair, fine line, wrinkle, or dark
spot isn't healthy, but there's nothing wrong with trying to look our
best—as long as it doesn't eclipse the more important things in life.

Your skin is the largest organ in the body, and it's also the one that
takes the biggest hit from the environment. The appearance of your
skin is directly related to your health as a whole. If you're filling your
body with processed foods, sodas, and other toxins, your skin will
show the results. If you're keeping toxins flushed out through cardiovascular exercise and plenty of water and providing your body's cells
with the phytonutrients present in fruits and vegetables, your skin will
also show those results.

In choosing what to put on your skin, here are some basics:

+ **Cleanse daily and gently.** Makeup and our environment fill
the pores in your skin with "dirt" of various types, regardless

of how carefully you choose the products you use. Using a gentle cleanser with tepid water every evening will help your skin breathe, heal, and refresh during the night. Don't leave your makeup on overnight.

- **Keep your skin moist.** Dry skin looks older and ages faster. Sunlight, heaters, air-conditioning, and makeup all dry out your skin. Using a daily moisturizer helps your skin stay healthier under all the insults it receives. Choose carefully based on whether your skin is naturally dry or oily.

- **Consider the use of retinol.** Many antiaging skin products now contain retinol, and it's one ingredient that has solid antiaging science behind it. Some skin may be quite sensitive to retinol. If you choose to use it, you may need to build up to daily use gradually.

What you keep *off* your face is more important than what you put *on* your face. Or, more accurately, what you refuse to allow to get to your skin matters most. Anything that damages DNA makes your skin look older and age faster. Lots of toxins can do that: sunlight, tobacco, or even the excess insulin and blood sugar of diabetes.

Here are several things you can do to keep your skin looking vibrant and youthful:

1. **Stay hydrated.** Lots of water is essential to keep toxins flushed away from your skin and allow the skin's cells to remain plump and healthy. Alcohol, sodas, or caffeinated drinks don't count here. Why do you think many models and actresses constantly drink water?

2. **Don't smoke.** By the time they're middle-aged, tobacco users appear about ten years older than non-users. Smoking greatly speeds up the appearance of wrinkles, fine lines, and dark spots. Quitting will stop the damage and allow your skin to repair itself to some degree.

3. **Beware of ultraviolet rays.** I once interviewed a couple where the husband was a dermatologist and the wife was a psychiatrist. They had a love-hate relationship with sunlight; it damages skin but improves

one's mood. The bottom line: when outdoors for any significant period of time, cover up with loose clothing and a hat, or use sunscreen. Ultraviolet rays are more dangerous than the chemicals in sunscreen.

4. **Exercise regularly.** The extra oxygen flowing through your blood vessels from exercise is wonderful for your skin, as is the sweating out of toxins. Exercise also helps decrease the risk of obesity, diabetes, and heart disease, all of which are bad for your skin.

5. **Eat plenty of fruits and vegetables.** The antioxidants in fresh produce are the best ammunition your skin cells have to combat the DNA-damaging things they come in contact with every day. This is yet another reason why I take and recommend Juice Plus+. (Read chapter 17 for more information.)

6. **Smile—a lot.** Research demonstrates that people who are smiling look significantly younger than people who aren't.[7] It takes fewer facial muscles to smile than it does to frown. You can actually improve your mental health by choosing to smile whether you feel like it or not. And smile wrinkles are so much more attractive than frown lines.

Investing in expensive antiaging products, dermatology procedures, or plastic surgery may help you look or feel a little younger. But no investment will pay off more than a pair of running shoes, some fruits and veggies, and a simple facial cleaning wash. And don't forget the smiles—they're free!

How to Stay Younger Longer

I'm not a fan of the antiaging industry. That's not because it's wrong to want to stay younger longer. And it's not even because some of the treatments and products recommended may have small positive benefits. It's because people spend so much time, money, and energy focused on things that may make a 1 percent difference in their health and longevity while ignoring more important things that will make an order-of-magnitude difference.

We know, for example, that growth hormone decreases as people get older. So does estrogen, DHEA (dihydroepiandrosterone) levels, and many other hormones. We know that the telomeres, the bits of DNA on the very ends of your chromosomes, get shorter as we age. We know that certain vitamins, minerals, or extracts from certain fruits and vegetables can stabilize those bits of DNA.

But what nobody has ever been able to do is stop the aging process. Nobody has been able to prove that an expensive program of hormones and other products will extend your healthy years any more than a seriously healthy lifestyle. Your "fountain of youth" is no farther away than your own home and the choices you make every day.

You can't stop the clock, biological or otherwise, but there are many things you *can* do to slow down the effect of time on your body, mind, and soul. In many ways you really are only as old as you feel.

How many of these stay-young practices do you do on a daily basis?

+ *Exercise.* There is probably no other single lifestyle factor as powerful for slowing the aging process as regular physical exercise. Our bodies were made to move. Physical exercise is one of the strongest ways to protect your body from disease and disability.[8] Not only that, but it also prevents aging in your brain.[9]

+ *Don't smoke.* The average middle-aged smoker has a physiological profile that's ten to fifteen years older than someone the same age who doesn't smoke. Countless studies show that smoking makes you age faster. The good news? The aging will slow down as soon as you put down the cigarettes.

+ *Stay mentally active.* Brain cells need exercise, too, throughout your life. Mental activity even helps lessen the inflammation that may be a cause of at least some dementia. Learning something new, reading, playing mental games such as crosswords or Sudoku, playing music—such mental exercise will keep your brain younger longer. Research here is a little controversial, but on balance the evidence is convincing.

+ *Nurture close relationships.* Studies document that loneliness is bad for your health.[10] Staying connected with people who care about you and whom you care about, such as children and grandchildren, a loving spouse, or young people you mentor, helps give you a reason for living. There will only be a few people around your deathbed. Nurture connections with those you will want around you as you get older.

+ *Choose a positive attitude.* People who stay healthy into old age are almost always happier in general than those who develop illness and disability. Which is the cause and which is the result? That's hard to determine, but what matters is positive emotions, which help counteract the effects of stress on aging. When seniors maintain a positive attitude, they realize a powerful benefit to their health.

+ *Get over grudges quickly.* Bitterness makes a person look and feel shriveled and old. A lack of forgiveness eats away at our physical, emotional, and spiritual health. Keep a short account of wrongs, and learn to let them go. Think of a miserable elderly person you know; don't let that kind of bitterness develop a permanent hold on *your* mind.

+ *Follow peace.* Stress wears you out physically, emotionally, and spiritually. Peace is not the absence of stressful elements in your environment but the inner calm that comes with security and maturity. Make a determined effort to learn ways to manage your stress. Ultimately Jesus, the Prince of Peace, is the answer at any age.

Perhaps you're disappointed that I haven't provided you with a list of products or supplements to combat aging. You may think the items I've listed here won't make that much of a difference. These items don't make for flashy headlines, but they are by far the biggest determinants in how you age, and how well you age. Nothing can do nearly as much to keep you younger longer than this kind of living.

This side of heaven, each of us will one day grow old and die. Let's determine to make every day count along the way.

FINISH WITHOUT REGRETS

Imagine yourself ten, twenty, or thirty years from now. How will you look back on your life? What will you wish you had done? How will you wish you had lived? What will you regret *not* having done?

One of the saddest statements anyone can make is, "What might have been?" None of us is likely to go through life without having at least some regrets. But how much better to live proactively so as to be able to look back and say, "I learned. I grew. I finished well."

Here are a few things you can do to help yourself finish without regrets:

+ **Care for your physical health.** That's one reason you're reading this book. Good for you! Once lost, health can be difficult to regain. Every positive choice you make today will have a greater impact than the same choice made in the future.

+ **Live your life fully.** Don't worry too much about what other people think. Invest in yourself, and follow your dreams.

+ **Learn to love well.** We've said it several times: investing in personal relationships is one of the best investments you can make. Children, parents, spouse, friends—learn to love them extravagantly and wisely.

+ **Remember your heart.** Even if you lose your physical health, your inner being can be alive and well. Be sure you're nourishing your soul regularly with fulfilling activities, healthy people, and a relationship with God.

Remember that imaginary talk with your nineteen-year-old self we mentioned in the last chapter? You can't have *that* talk, but there's another talk you can have. When you imagine yourself ten, twenty, or thirty years older than you are right now, what do you think your older self would tell the self you are right now? Have *that* talk today. Would the older "you" tell yourself to do anything differently?

Well, what are you waiting for?

A FEW QUESTIONS

Q: Do antiaging skin products really work?

A: Perhaps not. A Consumer Reports review of antiwrinkle creams summarized their evaluation by saying, "Alas, we were underwhelmed."[11] Doesn't make you feel very encouraged, does it? Products containing retinol may be helpful. Otherwise, you'll get the most mileage from keeping your skin healthy from the inside.

Q: How does God look at aging?

A: Very kindly. He's well able to use you in your senior years. Remember, Moses didn't begin his primary life's work until he was eighty. Psalm 92 says, "They will still bear fruit in old age, they will stay fresh and green" (v. 14). God has promised, "Even to your old age and gray hairs I am he, I am he who will sustain you" (Isa. 46:4). A relationship with God provides a hope for eternity that will become ever more precious as your life here grows shorter.

YOU AND YOUR DOCTOR

Chapter 14
VISITING YOUR DOCTOR

S HANNON WAS SCHEDULED to undergo an unpleasant but necessary outpatient procedure. She was at the surgery center on time, having carefully followed all the preoperative instructions.

"Do you have your medication list with you?" asked the admissions nurse.

"Yes, I do," Shannon replied, and she quickly tore a sheet out of her notebook. She had come prepared.

A moment later the nurse burst out laughing. "And just how often do you take this cake mix, eggs, milk, and sugar? And how much do you take?"

Soon Shannon was laughing too. Instead of her medication list she had handed the nurse her shopping list!

Sometimes you do have to laugh at the complicated and challenging journey that is your health care. Among the professional relationships you'll have during your lifetime, the relationship between you and your doctor is one of the most important. There's nothing I enjoy more as a physician than developing and maintaining an ongoing relationship with the women I have been privileged to care for.

A long-term relationship with a primary doctor you know and trust and who knows you well can be one of your best assets in staying healthy. Unfortunately, that doesn't happen very often in twenty-first-century America. Today you're more likely to receive your medical care from a group of physicians, see more specialists, and deal with many different health-care institutions. Some of the choices you may have made for yourself in the past regarding your health care now seem to be made for you. Many women find these changes frustrating, impersonal, and negative.

These same changes make it all the more important for you to take charge of your own personal health care. Many of the earlier chapters in this book focused on helping you take charge of your health, and now it's time for you do the same with your health care. After all, it's *your* life, health, and health care we're talking about. No doctor, hospital, government institution, or insurance company will ever care as much about you as you do.

COMMUNICATION IS KEY

Doctors are people too. And so are nurses, physical therapists, X-ray technicians, nurse practitioners, physician assistants, medical assistants, social workers, and all the other members of the health-care team you may come in contact with. As with most people, they usually respond best to clear communication, respect, and honesty. Every person I know who cares for patients in a health-care setting chose that field because they wanted to help people in some way. And your doctor undoubtedly wants to help you too.

But because doctors are people, it also means they're human. There are a few bad doctors who lie and cheat and take advantage of people when they're vulnerable. Even good doctors can have a bad day every now and then, personality-wise. Most don't have a photographic memory, and none knows all there is to know about science and medicine. And they certainly don't know all there is to know about you.

Health Tip
Doctors are people too. Most respond best to clear communication, honesty, and respect. And remember that even good doctors can have a bad day.

You'll get the most out of interactions with your doctor if you see you and your doctor as partners working together to make the best decisions regarding your health and health care. You both have important roles to play. Your doctor may be the professional, but she can't do things for you, and she can't know what's going on with you unless you tell her. See your doctor as a critically important resource, but *you* remain in charge.

It helps to be prepared when you talk with your doctor. Think through what you want your doctor to know and what questions you want your doctor to answer. Most doctors are pressed for time, often through forces out of their control. They often can't converse with you as long as they would like. The better prepared you are, the more you'll get out of the time your doctor has available.

Before your doctor's visit, think through these points, and write them down if you think you'll have trouble remembering:

+ What symptoms you're having and when they began

+ Anything you've done on your own to try and help the issue, such as over-the-counter medication, dietary changes, and the like

+ Anything you're anxious or worried about, such as "Is this cancer?"

+ Anything you believe may be affecting your health in this area, such as stress, travel, sexual activity, and so on

+ Any specific questions you want answered

Being clear begins when you make your appointment. Tell the receptionist the primary problem for which you need to see your doctor. This will help them allot the appropriate amount of time for your appointment and also help the doctor be better prepared when she sees you.

Most doctors will only give you a short time to tell your story before they begin asking questions. That's the way they're trained. Be ready to tell your story in a minute or two. It's OK to have further questions, but get the main points out quickly. And be sure to state your main worry or problem up front. Bring notes with you if you need to. Don't wait until the end of the visit to bring up what you're most worried about, as your doctor may not have time to address it by that point even if she would like to.

Here's an example of how you might share your story with your doctor: "My last period was about six months ago. Since about that time, I've developed hot flashes that bother me at work and keep waking me up at night. And intimacy with my husband has become very uncomfortable. Red clover tea hasn't helped at all. I'm scared about taking hormones for these symptoms because my mother developed breast cancer, but I need something to help with these hot flashes."

Can you see how that both puts you in charge of your health care and helps your doctor know how she can help you? She will likely ask you a number of other questions, but you've presented the problem that the two of you will work on together. Based on the other details of your medical situation, she may suggest some further tests and may discuss with you why, in your particular situation, she believes hormone therapy would be safe and effective.

> **Health Tip**
>
> *Be ready to share your story with your doctor in a minute or two. Be sure to mention your biggest problem up front.*

Now it's your turn to ask questions. Asking questions is one of the most important things you can do to take charge of your health care. Ask for an explanation of anything you don't understand. As much as we doctors try to explain things, sometimes we fall into the trap of using medical language or assuming patients know things that they don't. Never, ever be afraid to ask.

Here are some specific questions you'll want to ask if your doctor doesn't bring them up:

+ What do you think is causing my problems? (Even if your doctor isn't sure, she should be able to discuss what she believes is going on with you.)
+ What will these tests tell us? How will it change what you recommend?
+ How soon should I realize a benefit from this medication? Are there any side effects?

Most of all, before you leave, make sure you know what you're supposed to do next, including when you should return.

PREPARE FOR YOUR APPOINTMENT

Especially if you're seeing a new doctor for the first time, whether a primary care doctor or a specialist, having certain information available will greatly increase the value of that first visit. Here are some things you'll want to do in advance:

+ **Know your medical history.** If your history is complicated, write it down in outline style and bring it with you. List any surgeries and their dates, any hospitalizations, and any ongoing medical illnesses with the date (approximate) when you were diagnosed.
+ **List your medications.** All of them! Over-the-counter, supplements, herbal remedies, vitamins, and those that need a prescription—write down every single one.
+ **Outline previous treatments.** For the particular problem you're bringing with you, outline any previous treatments you've tried and how you responded to them.
+ **Bring a copy of your medical records.** If your medical history is extensive, many doctors prefer to have you forward

your records in advance. Then they can review and summarize them for their own use before your visit, and that will make your time together more profitable.

+ **Know your family medical history.** Know any major illnesses your parents, siblings, or other close family members had or have, and at approximately what age they died (if not still alive). You may need to ask certain family members about these things if you don't already know.

Many medical practices now offer an online patient portal where you can input your health history prior to your visit. If this is available, use it. If not, at least bring this information with you.

Should you research your symptoms or illness online and bring printouts of your research to your doctor's appointment? Most doctors appreciate an informed patient. And the more you know, the better you can work together to manage your health and your health care. But your doctor isn't likely to have the time to read through a thick printout of Internet research. Instead, use your own research time to formulate questions to ask and discuss with your doctor, such as "Would this test be helpful?" or "Do you have experience with this medication?"

And while we're talking about Internet research on medical questions, let me urge you to be cautious. There are some wonderful medical websites out there. Most scientific research papers are available online, and patient groups have formed for almost every illness. But you also know that anyone can put anything on the Internet, whether it's true or not. Use good judgment when discerning the quality of the information you find. Is it from a respected scientific source? Or is it from a source that's trying to sell a product or make money? Reasonable people, including reasonable scientists and doctors, can disagree at times, but be especially cautious before you spend your money or base your decisions on something you read on the Internet.

WHEN YOU NEED TO FIRE YOUR DOCTOR

Not all doctor-patient relationships turn out well. One of the positive changes in the current health-care environment is that it's easier to change doctors now than it's ever been. Constantly doctor-hopping won't get you the best results for your health care, but if your relationship with your doctor is negative, it may be time to make a change.

It's probably time to fire your doctor if:

- **You don't like your doctor.** You're not looking for a best friend, but you should have a sense that your doctor is someone you can get along with, someone you feel comfortable telling your difficult secrets to, and someone who seems to understand you most of the time.
- **Your doctor doesn't like you.** Doctors are people too. Sometimes you can't escape the feeling that your doctor would rather see just about anyone else but you. Sometimes your personality and theirs just don't match. That happens.
- **You have difficulty trusting your doctor.** You need to be able to trust that your doctor has your best interests at heart and is telling you the truth. Sometimes doctors can be difficult to understand, but if he or she has lost your trust, it's time to go.
- **You don't get your questions answered.** Doctors have limited training in communication, but communication is a critically important part of your relationship with them. You absolutely must be able to ask any questions you have and feel reasonably satisfied that your doctor is giving you the best information they have at their disposal.
- **You can't get an appointment.** In today's health-care world some doctors are being forced to take on many more patients than they can reasonably care for. It may be difficult to find a doctor who's easy to see, but reasonable access is worth considering when deciding whether your doctor deserves to be fired.
- **Money is a closed subject.** Your doctor may not personally know the cost of treatments they suggest, but they usually have a general idea. They should also have someone available who can find this out for you if necessary. If they're not willing to discuss the financial aspects of your care, find a doctor who will.
- **Your doctor doesn't want you to get a second opinion.** You don't need your doctor's permission to seek a second opinion

if you are facing a challenging medical issue. Any reasonable doctor will understand your desire for another opinion and welcome your choice to seek one. The only exception should be a life-threatening emergency.

+ **Your doctor won't discuss other options.** Your own investigation may uncover alternative treatments, supplements, or research about your condition that your doctor hasn't talked about. You should feel free to discuss these options with them. They may or may not have an opinion or further information on the issue, but they should be willing to talk about it.

+ **Your doctor won't accept your decision.** It's your body, your life, your pocketbook, and your health. If you refuse to go along with a treatment your doctor recommends, they also have the right to fire you as their patient. But in most cases, you should be able to come to a mutual understanding about how to proceed.

+ **You just want to.** Truthfully you don't need a specific reason to change doctors. Sometimes you can't put your reason into words. If things just aren't a fit, it's OK to make a change.

If you find you need to change doctors, do so politely. If you request a copy of your medical records yourself, the law allows your doctor's office to ask you to pay for that copy. Once you establish a relationship with another physician, signing a release of medical information will allow them to obtain a copy of your medical records, usually without cost to you.

> **Health Tip**
>
> *If you can't trust, don't like, or strongly disagree with your doctor, it may be time for a change.*

CARING FOR YOUR MEDICAL RECORDS

The days when a few scribbled notes in undecipherable handwriting were considered adequate medical records are long over. Vital personal information regarding your health and sensitive information about some of the most intimate details of your life are recorded either on paper or electronically at any doctor's office, hospital, or other place where you've received medical care.

Your medical records legally belong to your doctor or hospital, but that doesn't mean you can't and shouldn't care about them. There has been some talk about changing the ownership of medical records so they belong to the patient, but that probably won't happen in the near future, if at all.

There are two big reasons you should care about your medical records. The first involves your own health. The accuracy and completeness of the medical record provides your future doctors or health-care providers with important documentation on previous treatments or procedures, your response to them, and other information important in managing your future health.

The growth of electronic medical records was supposed to make medical care safer and more efficient. If all your providers have access to the same accurate and complete health information about you, duplicate tests might be avoided, mistakes might be prevented, and treatment decisions could be more appropriate.

But the reality is far from that ideal. Progress is being made, but the challenge of making the computer systems of doctor's offices, hospitals, laboratories, and pharmacies talk with each other has proven an enormous task and one that no one anticipates will be complete for years to come. Plus, just because something is computerized doesn't guarantee it's more accurate or more helpful. For example, many medical software programs use drop-down menus and check-lists that make your doctor's ability to record your unique story very challenging.

So, what can you do? If your doctor or hospital offers an online patient portal, make full use of it. Enter your medical information personally upfront, and update it as necessary. If the portal allows you to review your doctor's notes or test results, do so. Hopefully you'll find everything is accurate, but make a note of anything you have a question about, and ask for a correction to be made or an addendum added.

The other reason you should care about your medical records is the problem of medical identity theft. Your medical record is worth a lot more to hackers than your credit card number. Criminals can use such information to fraudulently bill Medicare or other insurance companies, purchase medications or medical equipment to resell, or otherwise make significant profit. The health-care field has been slower than many other industries to adopt computerization, and cybersecurity for health care has only recently become a priority.

Any health-care entity, whether hospital, doctor's office, laboratory, or some other entity, that obtains your personal or health information is legally obligated to protect it and to notify you if they become aware of any breach in that protection. Such breaches have, unfortunately, become increasingly common. One recent statistic reveals that 29.3 million patient health records were compromised by some form of data breach between 2009 and 2013.[1] I'm one of that number myself. Although no harm may come to the majority of individuals whose data has somehow been compromised, the possibility is nothing to take lightly.

While the responsibility for protecting your health information rests with your doctor, hospital, or other health-care facility, there are some things you can and should do to protect yourself or lessen your risks should your information become compromised:

- **Regularly check your credit report.** Fraudulent medical billing may eventually show up as a negative finding on your credit report, alerting you that something may be amiss and giving you an opportunity to investigate and make corrections.

- **Go online.** If your doctor or hospital offers an online patient portal, use it. And check it after any contact with the health-care system.

- **Consider credit protection.** This won't prevent hackers from taking your medical information, but it can limit your personal damages should financial implications occur. Companies offering such protection (such as LifeLock and others) also often provide assistance in dealing with your stolen information should a problem develop.

- **Keep your own records.** Names of doctors and hospitals, dates, medications, procedures, diagnoses—keep this information where you keep other important papers. You may never need it, but it helps to be prepared.

I wish I could be more reassuring about the security of your health information. Things are certainly better now than they were a few years ago, but there are still significant risks.

None of this should prevent you from being honest with your doctor. It may be embarrassing to tell her about your abortion, your family history, your struggle with substance abuse, or some other personal information, but tell her anyway. The risks of hiding such information from your doctor are too great. It's not worth it.

Has Your Doctor Made a Mistake?

Providing medical care is complex. Doctors are human. And when human beings do complex things, errors can happen. Many safeguards are in place to limit the impact of human error in providing health care, but it can still occur. Every doctor I know, including myself, has made an error. Most of them don't result in any damage to you and might be something as simple as writing *left* instead of *right* when describing an ovarian cyst, or overlooking a previous surgery on your medical history.

If you're concerned your doctor has misunderstood something you told her, overlooked a test or its results, or made some other "mistake," speak up. Remember, it's *your* health and your health care. Most of the time your doctor will be glad you spoke up and made things clear or alerted them to something they may have overlooked. It's one of the very powerful aspects of asking questions.

If you still have concern that aren't being addressed, you have the right to request a copy of a specific test result or your entire medical record. I have some patients who request a copy of every test result they receive, not because they believe there's a problem but just to have the information. And that's OK.

And remember, you can always get a second opinion. That's one of the *good* things about our system of medical care.

Clear communication, respect, and honesty will go a long way in making your relationship with your doctor a positive one. Remember to ask questions. More power to you!

A Few Questions

Q: What if I believe my doctor has committed malpractice?

A: If you believe a medical error has caused you or a family member serious harm, first, get the best medical care you can. If you want to seek care from another physician, do so. Not all mishaps are medical malpractice. Some complications are an understood risk of your particular medical condition or the treatment you decided on. Before you decide to sue your doctor for malpractice, consider how long most lawsuits take (usually years). Decide in advance what you're after. Is it money? An apology? Answers about what happened? Sometimes you can get what you need without a lawsuit. If not, be prepared for an emotionally draining journey with many long waits and frustrations. The majority of lawsuits end without the patient getting any money.

Q: Can I ask my doctor for a specific test, medication, or surgery?

A: Sure you can. Direct-to-consumer advertising has become big business, and many patients now ask about specific brand-name medications or treatments. Be aware that the most effective, least expensive, or best treatment for you may not be the one you see advertised. Marketers get their money from higher prices on the medical goods they promote. But it's also possible that what you ask your doctor for may be a good choice for you. Many doctors are happy to provide what you ask for if it's reasonable.

Chapter 15
DO YOU REALLY NEED THAT TEST?

DOES ANYONE ENJOY medical tests? Not anyone that I know. Who enjoys being poked and prodded, stuck with needles, exposing their most intimate parts, or having their breasts squeezed? The hassle and discomfort are enough to make any woman want to limit tests to those that are absolutely necessary.

And there's the cost factor. If you pay for your medical screening tests out of pocket, it's more likely you won't do them at all. That's why many health insurance programs cover recommended screening tests at little or no cost to you. Even if you aren't paying for them directly, the cost of those screening tests is built into what you pay for health insurance. And if your employer or the government is paying for your health insurance, it still comes out of your pocket in some way (but more about that in the next chapter).

How do you go about choosing which screening tests to have? Many national organizations have their recommendations to make, and your doctor has his or her own philosophy on what tests to order. This chapter will help you understand the reasons why some screening tests are recommended and others aren't, and help you make your own decisions on whether or not to have those tests.

Remember, it's your body, your health, and your health care. *You* remain in charge.

KNOW YOUR TESTS

Risk factor, screening test, and diagnosis—these are concepts that can be confusing, and understanding the differences will help you make informed decisions about medical tests.

A *risk factor* is a characteristic that makes it more likely you have or will develop a given disease compared with someone without that characteristic. Being female increases your risk for breast cancer; women get breast cancer about ten times more frequently than men do. Smoking increases your risk of lung cancer. Being overweight increases your risk of diabetes. If your mother developed breast cancer, especially before menopause, you have a higher risk of developing breast cancer also. And so it goes.

Screening tests are conducted to determine whether your risk for a given condition is greater or less than some other woman of your age and general characteristics. After a positive screening test, other tests are required to provide an actual diagnosis. An ideal screening test would:

+ Be able to detect the condition before you develop symptoms
+ Be relatively inexpensive
+ Not be associated with significant health risks
+ Be reasonably accurate, detecting most or all cases of the disease in question without detecting lots of unrelated and unimportant conditions
+ Detect a condition for which early treatment is available

A blood test for diabetes in a fifty-year-old woman who is overweight is a good screening test. It's accurate, inexpensive, and easily detects the disease before symptoms are present. Treatment for diabetes or prediabetes is readily available and effective.

A PET scan for Alzheimer's disease in a sixty-year-old women with occasional "senior moments" is a poor screening test. It's expensive, has some real risks, and isn't that good at detecting the condition. Plus, there are few, if any, treatments shown to be effective in stopping the disease. As you might imagine, for a disease such as Alzheimer's, scientists are trying to develop better screening tests that can more accurately and inexpensively detect the illness prior to symptom development, as well as develop effective ways to slow progression of the disease.

Recently CAT scans of the lungs in women who have smoked for a number of years have been recommended as a good screening test. The expense of the test has decreased, it's better than a simple X-ray at picking up cancer, and earlier treatment of lung cancer allows for longer survival and occasionally a cure. If you're a smoker or a former smoker, this is something you should talk with your doctor about.

There's plenty of debate among scientists, doctors, and economists over whether certain screening tests should be recommended, and for whom. Different medical organizations regularly publicize their interpretation of the number crunching and make pronouncements about who should or shouldn't have what tests. Sometimes these recommendations are quite controversial, such as the recent debates about when and how often women should receive mammograms or the value of PSA (prostate-specific antigen) testing for men over age fifty.

Most of these recommendations are strongly based on cost effectiveness—how expensive the screening test and any possible follow-up tests would be versus how much longer someone might live if the disease were found early and they received effective treatment. For this reason, I look very skeptically at the recommendations these organizations make. Such a broken system is the only one we have to work with, but how much better to educate yourself and make your own informed decisions on what screening tests you receive.

Concerning *diagnosis*, a screening test rarely provides one. It only comes from more definitive tests, such as further blood tests or a biopsy. For example, most women with an abnormal mammogram won't have breast cancer; the only way to find out is with further tests.

Those further tests also create some controversy over what screening tests to recommend. Having a breast biopsy, for example, is not risk-free. There's the anxiety that comes from waiting for the results, the pain and expense of undergoing the biopsy, the small risks of the procedure itself, and the potential—faced by many women—of undergoing such a procedure when breast cancer may not be present.

Now that you understand more about what screening tests do and don't do, let's talk about some of the commonly recommended screening tests so you can decide for yourself whether to have them done. Please note that in the United States, the US Preventive Services Task Force (USPSTF) offers recommendations on many screening tests.[1] My recommendations here may or may not be similar to what the USPSTF suggests.

PAP AND/OR HPV TESTS

I will always remember Mary, a forty-three-year-old woman I met in the emergency room when I was an ob-gyn resident. She hadn't seen a doctor in years, and I don't think she'd ever had a Pap test. Her family finally brought her in when she became too weak from prolonged vaginal bleeding.

Mary had late-stage cervical cancer. She died less than three weeks later. If she'd only had a Pap test sometime within the previous five or ten years, we would likely have been able to find and treat the cancer before it killed her.

A Pap test includes nothing more than scraping cells from the outer portion of the cervix and then looking at them under the microscope. Pap tests aren't perfect, but they do save lives. Cervical cancer rates have dropped dramatically since Pap tests became available. And because in our culture a majority of women have Pap tests, most abnormalities are treated long before they ever become cancer.

We can now detect the specific strains of the human papillomavirus (HPV) that cause cervical cancer—so-called high-risk HPV. In young women, this virus is often eliminated by the body's immune system over time. Finding and treating every case of HPV in young women might prevent cervical cancer, but it would also lead to many unnecessary biopsies and surgeries. Cervical cancer is usually very slow-growing. That's why HPV testing is only recommended for young women if the Pap test is abnormal. If an older woman still has HPV present, it usually means her immune system has been unable to eliminate the virus. That's why gynecologists recommend all women over age thirty have HPV testing done also.

There's a somewhat complicated algorithm gynecologists use to decide what happens after a woman has an abnormal Pap test or tests positive for high-risk HPV. Briefly, if the abnormalities are mild, your doctor may choose to simply repeat the test in six months, giving your body a chance to take care of things. If the abnormalities are more concerning or they persist, a colposcopy is done. For this procedure, a filtered light and magnifying lens are used to view the cervix, usually after placing a vinegar-like solution on the cervix that makes abnormal areas easier to detect. Any abnormal areas are biopsied to provide a specific diagnosis. Treatments such as freezing or LEEP (using a wire with an electric current to remove abnormal cells) usually prevent the HPV-associated abnormal cells from continuing to progress toward cancer.

Should You Have a Pap and/or HPV Test? Yes.

- *If you're age twenty-one to thirty and have had sex at least once, get a Pap test at least every three years.*
- *If you're over thirty, get a Pap and HPV test at least every five years.*
- *Have more frequent tests done if any of your tests are abnormal or if your doctor believes you may be at risk for HPV-associated abnormalities.*

MAMMOGRAMS

To a woman, *breast cancer* are two of the most feared words in the English language. There's lots of emotion connected with this disease, and some well-known women who developed breast cancer have publicized breast cancer well. A mammogram—simply an X-ray of the breasts—is still the best screening tool available, though it has many downsides.

Mammograms clearly detect many breast cancers while they're small and are usually treated more easily. What's more controversial is how often that early detection and treatment saves lives. Large research studies have evaluated death rates from breast cancer before and after a mammogram-screening program was implemented in a given country, and the results are difficult to interpret.

How often women should have mammograms and at what age they should begin is somewhat controversial. Before menopause, a woman's breast tissue is more dense, which makes interpreting a mammogram more difficult. Women under age fifty are also less likely to develop breast cancer. Doing mammograms every year only detects a few more early cancers than doing them every two years. Because of these factors, some scientists recommend women only have mammograms done every two years and that they begin at age fifty. Following this plan would prevent some unnecessary breast biopsies, but it would also miss some cases of early cancer.

Is radiation with mammograms a concern? Mammograms use a very small dose of radiation, but repeated mammograms over a number of years might add up to a minimally increased risk of cancer in some women. Switching to MRIs would be very expensive and time-consuming and might carry its own risks. The ideal screening tool for breast cancer is still out there, and studies are ongoing.

I tell my patients that doing yearly mammograms beginning at age forty saves lives. Not all doctors agree. But if you're a woman with breast cancer, wouldn't you want to know as early as possible? You'll have to make your own decision about mammograms, and your doctor should respect your decision.

When it comes to the actual procedure, we can all agree that it's not fun to get squeezed—so why not do something to spice up the experience? Look for a women's center that specializes in mammogram services. Get together with a couple girlfriends and make your appointments for the same time. Then go do something special together afterward.

One of the most important factors in how a radiologist interprets your mammogram is whether any changes are seen year to year. If possible, obtain your mammograms from the same location each year. If not, ask for a copy of the films from your previous mammograms (either digital or true film) to give to your new radiologist. This will allow them to provide a more accurate and helpful report.

We're talking here about screening mammograms. More extensive diagnostic mammograms are done if the screening mammogram is abnormal or if you or your doctor found a breast lump that doesn't go away. If a mammogram is abnormal, there are several ways to obtain a diagnosis: fine-needle aspiration, core needle biopsy, or open breast biopsy. The details of the abnormality seen on your mammogram often determine which method is recommended.

Should You Have a Mammogram? Yes.

- *Get a mammogram every year beginning at age forty.*
- *Begin earlier if your mother or sister developed early breast cancer.*
- *Get a mammogram anytime you or your doctor feel a breast lump that doesn't go away.*

COLONOSCOPY

Colon cancer ranks third among cancers women experience, right after lung cancer and breast cancer. Death from colon cancer is almost completely preventable. Not smoking and eating plenty of vegetables will decrease your risk. The American Cancer Society reports that long-term survival is possible for about 90 percent of those diagnosed with early-stage disease, compared with about 10 percent for those with late-stage disease.[2] That's why early detection is so important.

Several tests have been developed to detect colon cancer early—or, better yet, detect precancerous polyps in the colon before they develop into cancer. Among these are tests for blood or abnormal DNA in stool, barium enema, virtual colonoscopy (using CAT scan), sigmoidoscopy, and colonoscopy. Any of the tests other than colonoscopy may have a place in screening, but if anything abnormal is detected, a colonoscopy would still be necessary. A colonoscopy also allows for a biopsy of any suspicious areas and the removal of polyps if they're found. So a colonoscopy is often three things in one: screening, diagnosis, and treatment.

The preparation for a colonoscopy is the worst part of the experience. You'll be asked to limit yourself to clear liquids for about twenty-four hours prior to the test. You'll need to drink a solution, such as GoLYTELY or SUPREP, to evacuate all material from your colon. That means a lot of trips to the bathroom for one evening, but if your colon isn't clean, your doctor won't be able to adequately view all areas.

The procedure itself takes only a short time. And if all is well, you won't have to worry about it again for ten years.

Should You Have a Colonoscopy? Yes.

- *Get a colonoscopy every ten years beginning at age fifty.*
- *Get one done earlier or more frequently if you have colon disease or a family history of colon cancer.*
- *I recommend against the other tests for colon cancer unless you have a medical condition that makes a colonoscopy unsafe.*

BONE DENSITY

Osteoporosis may not be as deadly as heart disease or breast cancer, but it is common, painful, expensive, and disabling. And there are effective ways to slow down the bone loss of osteoporosis and limit the associated pain and disability.

Simple tests of bone density in a woman's heel or wrist have been popular and inexpensive. Unfortunately those tests can't accurately predict the bone density at a woman's spine or hip—the places where the most problematic osteoporosis-associated fractures occur. DEXA (dual energy X-ray absorptiometry) has become the standard because it can directly measure bone density at the most important locations and find osteoporosis before fractures occur.

DEXA screening is easy, painless, quick, and accurate. While you lie on a table, the DEXA scanner arm moves above your body, taking computerized measurements of the density of your bones. A well-tested computer program prints out specific measurements of your bone density at each of several vertebrae (bones in your back) and of your hip bones.

Health Tip

DEXA screening T score:
- *1 to -1: normal*
- *-1 to -2.5: low bone density*
- *Below -2.5: osteoporosis*

Your DEXA screening report will likely spit out a bunch of numbers; your T score is the one to know. It indicates how your bone density compares with that of young, healthy women. Most women after menopause will have a T score below 0. The lower or more negative the number, the lower your bone density.

If your T score is normal or near normal, you're probably fine with exercise, enough calcium, and retesting in two years or longer. If your T score is lower or indicates osteoporosis, your doctor will likely recommend more frequent testing and possibly prescription medication.

As with all tests, DEXA machines can vary depending on the manufacturer, location, and other factors. If possible, obtain your regular DEXA scans at the same location. Then you and your doctor can have more confidence that any difference from one scan to the next is a true change and not an artifact of the testing machine.

Should You Have a DEXA Bone Density Scan? Yes.

- *Get a DEXA screening done approximately every two years beginning at age sixty-five.*
- *Begin earlier if you have other risk factors for osteoporosis, such as the use of steroid medications, kidney or liver disease, or other factors.*

CARDIAC SCREENING

Heart disease is the leading cause of death among women. In this brief overview, I only have space to address my perspective as a gynecologist regarding the numerous heart tests sometimes promoted for women with no symptoms. If you have significant risk factors for heart disease or any symptoms that may indicate heart disease, please follow your doctor's recommendations.

First, the easy news. If you're under age fifty, don't smoke, are not obese, and don't have high blood pressure or diabetes, it's very unlikely that you have heart disease. In such a low-risk category, you probably don't need any cardiac testing at all.

The challenge comes for those with an intermediate risk. Perhaps you have a strong family history of heart disease or you have high blood pressure. In the endnotes you'll find two online tools that can provide you with your risk for experiencing a heart attack in the next ten years.[3] You'll need to know your height, weight, and blood pressure. If you've had a blood lipid panel done (for cholesterol, triglycerides, etc.), entering these numbers can provide you with even more detailed information about your risks.

If you're not sure of your cardiac risk, talk with your doctor. Ask for help in figuring out your global cardiac risk score by some method (such as one of these online tools). If you're at intermediate risk, further testing may be appropriate.

> ### Health Tip
>
> *Your global cardiac risk score indicates your chance of having a heart attack or major heart disease over ten years.*
>
> - *High risk:* more than 20 percent
> - *Intermediate risk: 10 to 20 percent*
> - *Low risk: less than 10 percent*

Some appropriate tests at this stage include the well-known EKG, an echocardiogram (ultrasound of the heart), or coronary calcium score. This last test has received a lot of publicity, but it's not for everyone. It's only appropriate if you have an intermediate risk of heart disease in order to help determine whether you're actually at lower or higher risk.

If you have high blood pressure or diabetes, you definitely need cardiac testing. What type and how often will depend on your doctor's recommendations.

> ## Should You Have Cardiac Screening?
> ## Yes—If You're at Intermediate Risk.
>
> • *Find out your blood pressure and cholesterol levels first.*
> • *Determine your global cardiac risk score.*
> • *Consider additional cardiac testing.*

SKIN EXAMINATIONS

Most people don't worry much about skin cancer—but it can kill. More than sixty thousand people die of melanoma every year. And since all skin is visible, it pays to pay attention.

People with fair skin, those with a family history of skin cancer, or those who have skin damage from being in the sun are at significantly increased risk of all types of skin cancer. If that's you, you especially need regular skin exams.

Begin by knowing your own skin. Look at every inch of it. Part your hair. Use a mirror to look at hidden places. Get to know the color, moles, lumps and bumps, or dark spots. By the time you're about forty, it's a good idea to get in the habit of looking at your skin monthly. If you notice anything new or different, such as a changing mole or new bump that doesn't go away, ask your doctor about it.

A yearly skin exam by a dermatologist is a quick and painless way to avoid potential skin cancers. When found early, almost every skin cancer is curable. Such an exam takes less than fifteen minutes, and any suspicious areas can quickly be evaluated with a biopsy.

> ## Should You Have a Yearly Skin Exam by a Dermatologist? Yes, If:
>
> • *You're fair-skinned with any sun damage*
> • *You or anyone in your family has had skin cancer*
> • *You notice any suspicious or concerning spots*

YEARLY PHYSICAL EXAM AND BLOOD TESTS

Most doctors used to recommend that everyone have a yearly physical exam whether they needed it or not. However, those physical exams rarely discovered anything important. I suggest you think of each visit to your doctor as being for a specific purpose, whether that's to discuss symptoms or questions you have, a test you need ordered, or a prescription you need filled.

Even so, it's smart to ask yourself each year whether there's something you should be scheduling a visit with your doctor to discuss. Many women use their birthday to remind them to do this. If you're under forty, your visit becomes an opportunity to discuss contraception and obtain a Pap test if needed. If you're over forty, you may need to order your mammogram, review any menopausal symptoms you might have, or request other blood tests.

Doing a panel of blood tests when you don't have any symptoms isn't useful very often. While many doctors have a panel of blood tests they offer yearly, these tests aren't likely to find anything important unless you're having specific symptoms. However, a few blood tests make the grade as being important on some type of schedule. Here's my list:

+ Fasting lipid profile (total, LDL, and HDL cholesterol, triglycerides): every three to five years; more frequently if you have a family history of heart disease
+ Hepatitis C: at least once; every woman over fifty
+ Fasting glucose or hemoglobin A1c: every three to five years beginning at age forty to screen for diabetes; more often and earlier if you're obese, have other risk factors, or have a family history of diabetes
+ TSH (thyroid stimulating hormone): every five years starting at age forty to screen for thyroid dysfunction
+ Vitamin D: if you're over sixty-five, want to take supplements, or have nonspecific symptoms

There are many more tests you might consider, but be sure you understand what your doctor is looking for. Most of the time, the tests listed here will be sufficient unless you have other health risks.

A FEW QUESTIONS

Q: What about screening for ovarian cancer?

A: Ovarian cancer is a difficult disease to screen for. Pelvic ultra-sounds and CA 125 blood tests have been suggested as possible ways to screen for this terrible disease. But these tests can't distinguish well between ovarian cancer and other benign conditions, including the normal changes a woman's ovaries go through every month with ovulation. For the majority of women without symptoms, doing these tests routinely would subject them to unnecessary worry and surgery.

The situation is different, however, for women who have symptoms or a family history of ovarian cancer. Be sure to talk with your doctor if you're in this category.

Q: Can I request a test myself, without a doctor's visit?

A: There are some tests now being marketed directly to consumers, without needing a doctor's order. These include some DNA tests, HIV testing, or even some cardiac tests or body scans. It's difficult to make a blanket statement regarding all these tests. While some are good, many of these tests are primarily money-makers for those who promote them. Most important, remember that you are a person, not a number on a test result. If you do choose one of these direct-to-consumer tests, make sure to discuss the results with your doctor if you have any questions at all about the results. And such testing is no substitute for a conversation with your doctor about anything that concerns you.

Chapter 16

NAVIGATING THE HEALTH-CARE SYSTEM

HEALTH INSURANCE. OBAMACARE. Deductibles. Monthly plan premiums. Copays. Drug benefits. In network or out of network. Covered benefits. Out-of-pocket maximum. Employee cost-sharing. Subsidies. Individual mandate. You need a textbook just to understand the vocabulary! And by the time you read this, there may be several more code words used to describe the complexities of our twenty-first-century US health care system.

The system can seem big and impersonal. And it is. Nobody—not the government, not your insurance company, not your hospital, not even your doctor—can care more about you and your health than you do. And that's the bottom-line reason why you must remain in charge of both your health and your health care.

According to the World Bank, the United States spends over 17 percent of its gross domestic product on health care—more than any other nation on the earth.[1] Every nation's health-care system is different. While many of the principles outlined in this chapter will apply wherever you're reading this, the specifics apply to the system we have currently in the United States. Our system is messy, and it has both very good aspects and very bad aspects. The politics and economics involved can be quite confusing.

In this chapter I'm focused on just one thing: helping you make individual choices based on the realities of our system as it is today. We won't talk about health-care policy. We'll look at the way things are today and give you the tools you need to make it work for you.

Remember, you're in charge!

PREPARE FOR CHANGE

When your grandmother became seriously ill, her mother may have telephoned the family doctor and waited anxiously until he arrived at her home. My grandfather was one of those family doctors. His youngest daughter, my aunt, remembers sitting on his black doctor's bag while driving with him to make house calls on summer mornings.

Anyone with a sore throat got a shot of penicillin (once it became available). Health insurance didn't exist.

Today medical science expands exponentially every year, but providing the care that science suggests has also become much more expensive. The ways in which you as an individual receive and pay for that medical care can also change almost as rapidly as the science itself. Here are a few of the current trends our health-care system is wrestling with and how some people experience those changes:

+ **Personalized medicine.** We can know the details of anyone's genetic makeup within a matter of hours or a few days. That presents many challenges. How do we protect your privacy and prevent discrimination based on your genetic makeup? Knowing what's in your genes doesn't always translate into knowing what treatments will be more effective. Do you really want to know what diseases you might get in the future if there's nothing you can do about them? And how do you tell others in your family that they may have the same genetic "problem" you have?

+ **Doctor networks.** With the pressure to save money, many health insurance plans are tightening their networks of doctors and hospitals. Some people find that the doctors they had previously are no longer "in network." Finding a new doctor in your health insurance's network can be difficult. Some people find they have to travel a lot farther than they did before to receive care, even when there are good health-care facilities nearby.

+ **Doctor shortages.** This is a loudly debated topic in some health-care circles, and the reasons are complex. Medical training is long and expensive to both students and society, making it a lengthy process to increase the number of doctors available. Most larger cities are unlikely to have serious doctor shortages anytime soon, but it may be much harder for smaller or more rural areas to recruit adequate numbers of physicians. Some people are finding that this means longer waits for appointments or receiving more of their care from non-physicians, such as physician assistants or nurse practitioners. Your doctor probably has less time to spend with you than he might like.

+ **Health insurance changes.** The much debated Affordable Care Act is making health insurance available to some and more expensive for others. As health-care costs continue to increase, both insurance companies and employers are passing on more costs to consumers. This often means you'll pay for more of your health care yourself through deductibles and copayments. Insurance companies are also becoming increasingly sophisticated in controlling more of what health care they will or won't pay for.

+ **Focus on lifestyle diseases.** Best known among the so-called lifestyle diseases are those illnesses caused in whole or in part by obesity or tobacco use. This means more insurance companies and employers are offering financial incentives for such things as quitting smoking or enrolling in a weight-loss program. Healthy lifestyle messages are showing up in more places than ever. Some people find this intrusive. Others find it helpful for making necessary lifestyle changes to become healthier.

+ **New ways of providing health care.** "Cash only" clinics and physician practices that don't accept any health insurance are growing. Some provide basic services for a relatively small fee, perhaps less than an insurance copay. Others offer boutique services, such as unlimited physician contact and extended doctor visits for a monthly retainer fee. Also increasing in popularity are health-sharing ministries, where members contribute a monthly amount that is used to cover the costs of members' health-care needs. (There's more about these ministries later in this chapter.)

How you feel about these changes likely depends on your financial circumstances and where you live. Your political or religious views likely impact your thoughts on these matters as well. Now, what can you do in response?

KNOW THE COSTS

Through experience, most people have been trained to ask, "Does my insurance cover this?" Medicare, Medicaid, or your health insurer made the decisions, and most people followed along. Movies like *John*

Q highlight individuals fighting with the powers that be to get them to pay for a treatment that didn't fit within their guidelines. Things change, and current buzzwords in health-care policy include *safety*, *prevention*, and *quality*, which are admirable but often costly goals.

Somebody must pay for every bit of health care you receive. That's something most people don't think about. If you have Medicare, the government pays your doctor or hospital from a trust fund you paid into along with your employer. But that money isn't nearly enough. Other tax dollars have to be collected to keep the program going. If you're on Medicaid or receive other government assistance, people's taxes, including yours, are paying for the care you receive. And the costlier that care is, the fewer tax dollars are available for roads, police, schools, and the like. All government health programs are very expensive in that they take a significant portion of the money to pay for the bureaucracy to administer the program.

Then there's the private health insurance market. Private companies sell you or your employer a service whereby they collect money from you and others and then pay your doctor or hospital when you need care. The more that

> ### Dr. Carol Says...
>
> *"All health-care costs you in some way. Just because someone else is paying the bill today doesn't mean it's free."*

care costs, the more money they need to collect from you beforehand. And of course, the insurance company keeps some of the money to pay brokers, administrators, and shareholders.

The bottom line? All health-care costs you in some way. Just because someone else is paying the bill today doesn't mean it's free.

If you were paying for your health care from your own pocket, you'd ask quite different questions. You'd want to know how important a given test was, how successful a given treatment or medication would likely be in taking care of your symptoms, or whether there was a less costly alternative that would work nearly as well. And as you do when you need a car or furniture, you'd shop around.

You should do the same with your health care. Think beyond whether or not your insurance company will pay for a given test or treatment. Ask what to expect with anything your doctor recommends—questions like, How will this test change how you treat me? What do you expect to find out? Is a generic medication available that will do the same thing? Can I get this test done anywhere I choose?

Your doctor probably doesn't know the exact cost of the tests or treatments they recommend, but they usually have an idea of which are more or less costly.

And you can shop around. The same medication may cost less at a different pharmacy. The same blood test may cost half as much at a different laboratory. You may be able to get the same X-ray or MRI done a few blocks down the street and save significant money. If your procedure can be done in an outpatient facility, it's likely to cost a fraction of what it would cost in a hospital.

I don't believe cost should ever be the only or primary reason for recommending any given course of medical treatment. The most expensive option doesn't always give the best results. It pays to consider what kind of value you're getting for your health-care dollar, whether or not you're the one spending it directly.

NEGOTIATE MEDICAL BILLS

One December morning a couple years ago I became the patient instead of the doctor when I was awakened in the middle of the night by severe abdominal pain. As a doctor, I knew the tests I needed, and I couldn't do them on myself. So I reluctantly woke up my husband, and we proceeded to the emergency room.

Thankfully my problem wasn't serious. In a couple hours I was back home feeling much better. But my pain didn't stop there. I had no health insurance at that time—by choice. I was facing thousands of dollars in medical bills and a lot of angst. But by using the process I'm about to describe, I was able to reduce my medical bills by more than 60 percent.

First, you need to understand how traditional health insurance works. If you have health insurance, how much your doctor or hospital receives for taking care of you is determined by contract. You may be asked to pay a portion of those costs, but the amount your doctor receives is always less than the "list price" for that service—sometimes a lot less.

Let's take a hypothetical scenario. You schedule a routine follow-up visit with your doctor. She charges $150 for that visit. If you have health insurance, your doctor may have agreed with the insurance company to accept $80 for that visit, and that's all she will receive. Or it might be only $55. Besides writing off the difference, she'll also have to hire someone to send a bill to the insurance company and wait for a few weeks (or longer) to receive payment.

If you see the same doctor for the same visit but you don't have health insurance, your doctor will still charge $150. She can't charge you less without getting into serious legal trouble. She must charge anyone the same amount for the same service, whether or not they have insurance.

But there's nothing saying your doctor can't *accept* less than the original price she charged you. She does this every day when she accepts payments from insurance companies. (This is why some doctors no longer accept insurance at all.) And most doctors will accept less than the list price. The trick is knowing how to ask.

Some doctors, laboratories, or other health-care facilities will offer you a significant discount for paying in cash at the time of service, sometimes 50 percent or more. If you pay right away, the doctor and her staff don't have to spend time billing an insurance company, waiting weeks for payment, and then going back into their files and writing off the difference. If your doctor offers such a discount, take advantage of it.

What if you're not happy with the discount offered? How do you know how much to offer in payment if no discount is suggested? Here's where my three-step plan can save you tons of money.

1. **Get an itemized copy of your medical bill.** Whether it's a hospital, laboratory, emergency room, or doctor's office, ask for a printed copy of the bill that includes the five-digit CPT (current procedural terminology) codes for every service you received. (For example, 99213 is the code for a routine follow-up doctor's visit for a moderately complex problem, such as menopausal symptoms.)

2. **Research the fair-market price for each code listed.** Two free online services make such research quite easy: Healthcare Bluebook, available at www

.healthcarebluebook.com, and Fair Health Consumer, available at www.fairhealthconsumer.org. To use these tools, you will be asked to enter your zip code because accepted costs are different in different areas of the country. Then enter each five-digit code into the website form and make note of the suggested price. Consider getting prices from both sites, as they may differ.

3. **Make an offer.** Using your research to understand what a reasonable price is for the services you received, take your printout of these fair-market prices with you to the hospital or doctor's business office, if necessary. Your offer is likely to be taken seriously and may be accepted immediately. If not, it will at least be a starting point for a serious negotiation.

Using this process, I saved 62 percent on my medical bills from my emergency room visit that day. I know it will save you money, too, if you must pay for your health care yourself.

Please note that this process only works if you don't have traditional health insurance, Medicaid, or Medicare. It won't apply if you receive care at a clinic that already offers a sliding scale of charges or a boutique office that provides extra services for an up-front retainer fee. It will, however, apply to any hospital or emergency room visit, traditional laboratory or radiology services, and most physician's office visits.

Even better than negotiating payment after you've received care, you can also negotiate beforehand for planned medical services. Some hospitals, for example, post their cash prices for common procedures right on their website. If you're prepared to pay up front, you save the hospital or doctor's office a lot of money, and they'll likely pass on much of those savings to you. If you have several choices for where to get your medical care and you find that one or more won't discuss money with you up front, consider going elsewhere.

But going without health insurance is not a wise long-term solution. NerdWallet reports that more than half of all bankruptcies are due to unpaid medical bills, even among people who do have health insurance.[2] There are better ways to approach this, including the approach I now use for my own medical costs.

CHOOSE YOUR HEALTH INSURANCE

If you receive health insurance through your employer, you may have a limited number of options to choose from. Such group insurance, however, is usually less expensive than purchasing your own health insurance directly from an insurance company. However, the amount of your monthly premium is only one item to pay attention to. When choosing a lower-cost insurance plan, many individuals don't think much about the deductible or copays. You may end up spending thousands of dollars of your own money before your health insurance kicks in.

Your individual and family circumstances play a big role in what options work best for you. Prior to signing any health-insurance agreement, either with your employer or on an individual basis, here are some things you need to know:

+ The amount of your monthly premium
+ The yearly deductible (how much you're required to pay out of pocket before your health insurance kicks in); this may be as low as $500 or as high as $10,000 or more
+ The copay for doctor's visits, hospital visits, and so on (how much of those charges you pay yourself); this may be a dollar amount, such as $25 per doctor's visit, or a percentage, such as 40 percent of the charges
+ Whether other services, such as laboratory, X-rays, prescriptions, vision care, or dental care, are included or available for an extra cost
+ Whether preventive care is available at little or no cost; most health insurance plans are now required to provide certain preventive services at no cost to you
+ Whether it includes a maximum amount you pay out of your own pocket each year (made up of your deductible and copays)
+ What doctors, hospitals, or other health-care services are in network and whether or not your insurance will pay for any care you receive out of network
+ Whether or not the doctors you already see are in network
+ Whether there are financial incentives related to lifestyle behaviors; for example, are there extra costs if you're a smoker,

or do you get a discount if you sign up for and achieve a certain weight-loss goal?

+ How high-cost or experimental medical treatments are
handled

+ Whether you have a right to appeal if your insurance company declines to pay for care you need or desire

Wow! Reading that list is likely to make any woman's head spin,
especially those who are not used to thinking about health insurance
much. It's no wonder many people just sign up for the least expensive
plan offered without thinking about the consequences.

Some of these questions will be more important to you than
others. Perhaps you live in a more rural area or have a longstanding
relationship with one specific doctor. Whether a specific doctor is
in network may be the deciding factor for you. Perhaps you know or
suspect you'll need some significant medical care in the coming year
and you want to keep your out-of-pocket costs low. In that case, the
yearly maximum you could be asked to pay might be most important.

By now, you know how strongly I feel about encouraging you to
remain in charge of your health care. When choosing health insurance, I believe one of the best ways to do this is to choose a high-
deductible plan along with a health savings account (HSA). This
allows you to save money tax-free to pay your portion of medical
expenses, but it also provides health insurance to pay for unexpected
or expensive medical care. You own the HSA. The money accumu-
lates from year to year, is usually tax-free, and stays with you even if
you change employers or retire. Using your own HSA money to pay
for your portion of necessary medical care helps you pay attention to
value and to choose wisely. If you have the option of an HSA along
with a high-deductible health plan through your employer, I strongly
encourage you to consider this option.

HEALTH-SHARING MINISTRIES

Imagine how nice it would be to never have to worry about whether
your health insurance covers a certain treatment or whether or not a
certain doctor was in network. These are only a few of the benefits of
kicking the middleman of the insurance company completely out of
the relationship between you and your doctor. Members of Christian

faith communities can do just that and save significant money on medical bills by joining a health-sharing ministry.

Some people also object to the possibility that their health insurance dollars might be used to pay for services for others that they themselves find morally objectionable. Health-sharing ministries eliminate that possibility.

These ministries have been around for several decades but are becoming increasingly popular as health insurance premiums and deductibles increase. As of this writing, members of these ministries are exempt from any penalties that individuals without health insurance might incur under the Affordable Care Act.

Health-sharing ministries are not health insurance. There is no contractual obligation between you and the ministry for them to pay for your medical care. You retain the responsibility for paying for your health care. Each ministry is a voluntary group of Christians agreeing to make a monthly contribution for the purpose of sharing in each other's health-care costs. When a member receives medical care that costs above an agreed-upon amount, the ministry forwards money directly to the member for their use in reimbursing the doctor or hospital.

The monthly amount members of these ministries are asked to contribute is much less than the cost of traditional health insurance—often one-third or less. Costs are kept low for several reasons. These ministries are nonprofit and don't have to satisfy shareholders. Members agree to follow certain biblical lifestyle guidelines, typically including things such as abstaining from tobacco, engaging in sexual intimacy only with their spouse, and attending church services regularly.

These ministries also provide strong prayer support and encouragement when members face health challenges. Many report that this aspect of the ministry is the most valuable. Staff members may also assist in negotiating medical costs, thus saving both you and the ministry money.

If you're looking for a faith-friendly way to manage your health-care costs, save money, and be a blessing to others in the family of God, consider one of these three ministries. They share similarities, but each have their own guidelines:

+ Christian Healthcare Ministries: www.chministries.org
+ Samaritan Ministries: www.samaritanministries.org

+ Medi-Share with Christian Care Ministry:
www.mychristiancare.org

I am currently a happy member of one of these ministries. You need not face the financial challenges of receiving medical care alone.

A Few Questions

Q: How can I save money on my expensive medications?

A: In the United States, there are strict regulations controlling the production of generic medications. In almost all instances, they are the same quality as brand-name medications. Generic medications usually cost a lot less and do the same thing. If paying for medications is difficult for you, ask your doctor about the lowest-cost alternative that will treat your symptoms. And for brand-name medications, NeedyMeds, available at www.needymeds.org, provides information on many patient-assistance programs.

Chapter 17

EVALUATING AND USING SUPPLEMENTS

WALK INTO ANY grocery store, pharmacy, or specialty nutrition center, and you're likely to be overwhelmed with aisles of pills, powders, and liquid extracts. Turn on the TV or spend a few minutes looking for just about anything online, and you can't escape the fancy advertisements promoting the latest potions or products. The promises fall just short of guaranteeing miracle cures for anything that ails you. The *Nutrition Business Journal* reports that global sales for supplements top $100 billion each year—and continue to increase.[1]

Remember the talk-show host I mentioned in chapter 1 who is taking sixty pills a day, all of them supplements? She's not alone. I know an elderly couple that was spending hundreds of dollars each month on supplements while having difficulty paying for other necessary items such as food. I know an evangelist who travels with an extra suitcase just to carry his supplements and has his entire pantry at home filled with them.

If that $100 billion is making us healthier, we should celebrate. But this trendy spending may not be doing us much good, and in fact may be causing real harm. How do you make decisions on whether to use supplements, and which ones should you take seriously? Which ones are likely to provide value for your health dollar?

My summary: you don't need sixty pills a day to be healthy! There's absolutely no way anyone—doctor, scientist, nutritionist, pharmacist—can tell you what will happen when you put that quantity of foreign substances into your body. Here are some common-sense and scientifically sound ways to sort through the claims and the data and make appropriate decisions about what you put in your body.

BUYER BEWARE

A hundred years ago, you could purchase Mixer's Cancer and Scrofula Syrup to treat a whole host of ailments, or arsenic and mercury to cure syphilis. Those remedies may sound archaic to us in the twenty-first century. They do remind us, however, that just because something is natural, that doesn't make it either safe or effective. A hundred years from now, we may look back on many of both the "natural" and prescription remedies we use today and laugh.

Just like the snake-oil cures sold a couple centuries ago, the supplement industry today is governed by little or no regulation. Such regulation can be either helpful or destructive. I'm not a fan of the US Food and Drug Administration. We do, however, need to use science rather than hype to make decisions about what we put into our bodies. Anecdotes (stories about one person's experience) or small "studies" financed by a company promoting its own product don't convince me, and they shouldn't convince you either. Scientific research has its limitations, but it's still the best way to answer the question, "Is Product X both safe and effective?" The FDA is, right now, the best we have, and it doesn't control the supplement industry.

The promise of "natural" is strong. We all believe, rightfully so, that something originating from God's green earth is likely to be better for our health than something created in a man-made laboratory. Most of the time that's true, but not always. Remember mercury and arsenic? They were, and are, certainly natural. So are poison ivy and poisonous mushrooms. My point is not that prescriptions are always safe or a good idea or that natural is necessarily dangerous. Most of the time, natural *is* best. We must, however, be just as cautious with the natural remedies we choose as we are about any other medical treatment.

We can easily fall into the ditch on either side of healthy on this issue. On the one hand, our environment yields a food supply that probably has less nutritional value than in the past, even in fresh produce. Our stressful lives place extra demands on our physical bodies. Prescription and over-the-counter medications have risks and side effects, and they may be prescribed too often by many doctors. Those facts would seem to make nutritional supplements useful.

On the other hand, just because something is, or claims to be, natural, that doesn't mean it's safe. Many, if not most, herbal substances have side effects just as significant, or more so, than prescription medications. Drug-herb and herb-herb interactions can also be dangerous, even life-threatening. It's important to be suspicious of claims that seem too good to be true.

And then there's the money. If you want to know the truth, follow the money, right? With supplements being such big business, it's understandable that many entrepreneurs will use clever marketing techniques to get you to part with your money based on the hope that something they promote will make you feel better or keep you away from the "big, bad doctor." A company selling a supplement can legally claim just about anything they want as long as they don't directly claim to diagnose, treat, or cure a specific illness. Any other claim is fair game, and there's no one to stop them.

Before parting with your hard-earned money, ask these questions about any natural product or supplement.

Is this information reliable?

A company website or the label on a bottle is not enough in itself to satisfy the reliability test. The same information should be verifiable from independent sources who have nothing to gain by providing misleading information. Such other sources might include medical specialty organizations, such as the American College of Obstetricians and Gynecologists, research published in scientific journals, or government organizations. Above all, don't trust a product website without checking elsewhere for confirming information.

What kind of claims are being made?

If it sounds too good to be true, there's good reason to be skeptical. Be wary of products that claim to support the health of an organ, such as the ovaries or breast. Companies selling health supplements have found that such wording usually allows them to escape sanctions by the FDA, but those claims don't have to be supported by scientific research.

> **Health Tip**
>
> *Follow the money! If the information supporting a given supplement only comes from the company making money on the product, be very suspicious.*

Is this product likely to interfere with other medications or supplements I'm taking?

Natural or herbal supplements may frequently interact with both over-the-counter and prescription medications. You should discuss *all* products you take with your doctor. Your pharmacist may be an even better resource for evaluating any interactions. Medications used to treat diabetes, blood-clotting problems, or high blood pressure are especially prone to interactions with natural supplements.

Is this specific product safe and reliable?

Supplement manufacturers are not held to the same standards as pharmaceutical companies. Perhaps that's a good thing. But that lack of oversight can result in products that contain vastly differing amounts of active ingredients from what is presented on the label. They can even contain dangerous ingredients that aren't listed. Consumer Lab is a private company providing independent testing and evaluation of the quality and content of hundreds of health and nutritional products on the market. If you regularly use supplements, consider subscribing to this inexpensive and informative resource, available at www.consumerlab.com.

It would be nice if you could trust anything you heard or read and have someone else do the investigation for you. In a small sense, perhaps that's what the list of supplements I recommend later in this chapter can, in part, do for you. But remember, it's your health, your life, and your pocketbook. Being an informed consumer helps you stay in charge.

Choose Supplements Wisely

Ideally, we wouldn't need any supplements. God knew what He was doing when He created growing things—fruits and vegetables—as our food. (See Genesis 1:29.) A diet that is based on a variety of plant foods that are as fresh as possible should provide most of us with the nutritional elements we need for good health. God knew that when He created us and the earth around us.

Our life and world today, however, are far from how God originally intended things to be. Using nutritional supplements when necessary makes sense from this perspective.

Supplements can't make up for an unhealthy diet or lifestyle. The very name implies it—they're meant to *supplement* a healthy diet, not replace it. Most of our nutrients of every kind should come from the food we eat.

The list of nutritional supplements I recommend is relatively short. A product or supplement must pass a fairly rigorous test for me to believe it's safe, effective, necessary, and worth the money spent. Here are some useful criteria that help define what supplements deserve recommendation:

+ **Support from scientific research.** Is there good-quality, unbiased research supporting the benefits and safety of this product or supplement? We'll probably never have all the data we want for any product, but there needs to be some science backing any recommendation. Stories of individual people's responses don't help here. The best research involves large groups, preferably randomized and placebo-controlled. When such research is supported by independent investigators who have nothing to gain from the results, that research has more credibility. Check things out yourself, and don't rely only on the company trying to sell you anything to tell you everything.

+ **Plausible claims.** If the claims sound too good to be true, they probably are. The more wonderful the product claims to be, the stronger the scientific research must be to back up those claims before they're worth believing. You should demand to know what kind of specific outcomes people who use this product have experienced.

+ **It makes sense.** Sometimes something just works, and nobody really knows how or why. Most of the time, however, there should be some logical reason why a given supplement is useful for a specific reason. There are certain medical conditions where using certain supplements makes more sense than others. Simply throwing tons of pills or powders into your body each day is not wise. Know what you're taking and why.

> **Health Tip**
>
> *Be suspicious of product claims that sound too good to be true. The more wonderful a product claims to be, the stronger the research you should demand to back up those claims.*

+ **Quality of the specific product.** Not all multivitamins are created equal. At a minimum, look for the USP mark (which indicates the stamp of the US Pharmacopeial Convention) on any product you purchase. The USP sets quality standards

for many dietary supplements. Consider checking Consumer
Reports at www.consumerreports.org and/or subscribing to
Consumer Lab at www.consumerlab.com. If the product is
a pill or capsule you take orally, drop one in a glass of water.
If it doesn't dissolve in water over several hours, it's likely
to have difficulty dissolving and being absorbed in your GI
system.

These may be high standards, and sometimes they're difficult to
meet. But they're worth asking about any supplement you consider.

SUPPLEMENT RECOMMENDATIONS

Enough of the background and theory. If you've read the previous
portions of this chapter, I'm proud of you. You want to know what
I recommend, and I want you to know why. If you haven't read the
earlier portions of this chapter, I encourage you to do so now. Then
you'll understand why this list is what it is.

First, a word on phytonutrients. *Phyto* refers to the Greek word
for *plants*. Fruits, vegetables, and whole grains contain tens of thousands of nutrients in various classes. We know the health benefits of
many of these nutrients, such as antioxidants, carotenoids, flavonoids,
polyphenols, and more. There are many more of these nutrients that
we may not know anything about at all. And we know even less about
which nutrients need to be taken together and in what ratio to have a
maximum beneficial effect. Many researchers believe that phytonutrients in combination may be much more beneficial to health than any
one taken individually. That's all the more reason why getting your
nutrition from nutrient-dense food is usually the best.

Now for the list. Here are the supplements I can recommend to
my patients and to you.

Phytonutrient supplements

Few of us get the recommended nine-plus servings of fresh fruits
and vegetables daily. These supplements can help make up the difference between a healthy diet and what our body's cells need most
to remain healthy. Look for a product that's made from ripe, whole
fruits and vegetables. Among other benefits, these products contain
concentrated phytonutrients in the ratios and combinations God

built into nature. The downside is that these products aren't regulated, so investigate the company you purchase from.

Data is accumulating on the benefits of these supplements for general health in such areas as chronic inflammation,[2] immune system function,[3] and more. These and similar benefits are thought to decrease the risks of heart disease and other illnesses, and research is ongoing to document this.

Juice Plus+, available at www.juiceplus.com, is the phytonutrient supplement I'm most familiar with and can recommend, but there are others. Taking it with a full glass of water will help prevent any gastrointestinal side effects.

Fish oil/omega-3s

Hundreds, perhaps thousands, of studies have been done on fish-oil supplements. Much of the research supports the likely benefits of fish-oil supplements for cardiovascular health, especially for people with elevated triglycerides. Omega-3 supplements may help prevent, slow down, or even slightly reverse atherosclerosis. Research is less clear on its possible benefits for brain health, asthma, and other conditions. There is considerable debate among contemporary scientists on whether people without high blood lipids or heart disease can benefit from fish-oil supplements. If you choose to take them, 1 gram per day on days you don't eat fish is reasonable.

Inositol

This is one of the most exciting supplements I have encountered in recent years. A number of studies indicate that inositol improves ovarian function, especially in women with polycystic ovary syndrome (PCOS).[4] There are two forms of inositol—myoinositol and d-chiro-inositol. Both forms are helpful and may be best taken in combination for many women with PCOS.[5] Individually the myoinositol form is more effective for improving egg quality and ovulation rates, and d-chiro-inositol is more effective for improving the androgenic problems of women with PCOS. Two brands to consider are Pregnitude, available at www.pregnitude.com, and Chiral Balance, available at www.chiralbalance.com, or you can find generic options.

St. John's wort

Numerous research studies have demonstrated that St. John's wort is as helpful for mild to moderate depression as many prescription antidepressants, such as Prozac, Celexa, and Paxil. And it doesn't appear to lower sex drive as many antidepressants do. Some believe St. John's wort also helps with premenstrual syndrome and the mood swings some women experience with menopause. It's available in tea, liquid extract, or time-release capsules, and it may take three to four weeks to notice any improvement in symptoms. St. John's wort may interact with a number of other medications and supplements, so be sure to check with your pharmacist before taking it.

Multivitamins

If you take a phytonutrient supplement and eat a healthy diet, you almost certainly don't need a multivitamin. I can't point to any evidence that multivitamins improve people's health in general. In fact, the Iowa Health Study followed more than 38,000 women for twenty years and found that those who took vitamins died sooner than those who didn't.[6] One study of male physicians showed a decreased risk of cancer among those who took multivitamins.[7] Pregnant women, those who struggle to eat a healthy diet, or those with other specific medical problems may do well to take a vitamin supplement. If you do take a multivitamin, check the list of ingredients against any other vitamin supplements you may choose to take. Getting too much of certain vitamins—especially vitamins A, D, and K—can be dangerous.

Green tea

Green tea is less oxidized and closer to "natural" than black tea, and therefore it contains more antioxidants. Compared with powdered or bottled teas, brewed green tea maintains the most phytonutrients. Many studies show that long-term use is associated with a decreased risk of certain cancers, and mental alertness is increased in those who use it daily. The large Ohsaki study from Japan showed that women who drank green tea regularly had a decreased risk of dying from all causes and from cardiovascular disease specifically (though not cancer in this study).[8] One recent review concludes that regular tea drinking is associated with a decreased risk of stroke, diabetes, and depression.[9] While freshly brewed green tea may be the best, green tea extracts are likely to be similarly beneficial. Beware of the potential side effects of too much caffeine, including anxiety, insomnia, and calcium loss from bones.

Calcium/magnesium

The best place to get calcium is from your diet, such as from dark green leafy vegetables or dairy products. Take extra only if needed, and only under a doctor's recommendation. A number of studies indicate that calcium supplements, even 1,000 mg daily, may increase cardiovascular disease by increasing the calcium deposits in areas of atherosclerosis. Some women find a combined calcium/magnesium supplement to be helpful for symptoms of PMS or muscle cramps. If you're getting adequate calcium from your diet, taking supplements isn't likely to lessen your risk of osteoporosis. However, if you're taking any medication that increases your risk of osteoporosis, such as steroids, if you're drinking a lot of green tea, or if you already have osteoporosis, taking a supplement may be important. Women past the age of menopause need 1,200 mg of calcium daily from both food and supplements. Use with caution.

Vitamin D

The research on vitamin D could fill this whole chapter, and more. Who needs it, how much they need, and how vitamin D affects various areas of health is very controversial. We know it's necessary for strong bones. Inadequate vitamin D levels have been associated with just about any disease you can name, including diabetes, obesity, fertility and pregnancy problems, heart disease, cancer, and multiple sclerosis. The much bigger question is whether supplements of vitamin D improve your health in any of these areas.

I highly recommend having a vitamin D blood test before taking any vitamin D supplement. If your level is 30 ng/mL or greater, you don't need extra vitamin D. Women over age seventy usually need vitamin D supplements because of the difficulty they have absorbing it adequately from food and the extra help they need to maintain strong bones. If you need supplements, your doctor should monitor your blood levels periodically until they're stable. Don't overdo vitamin D; too much of this good thing can be dangerous.

Folic acid

Research overwhelmingly shows that adequate folic acid intake before and during the early weeks of pregnancy reduces the risk for specific birth defects, especially those affecting the brain and spinal cord. Women who are or who may become pregnant should start with

0.8–1 mg daily. That amount is commonly found in prenatal vitamins or can be taken individually. Those who have a personal or family history of such birth defects and those taking certain medications, such as anticonvulsants (for seizures), need significantly more folic acid. There's a long list of other illnesses that folic acid has been recommended to help, including heart disease, breast cancer, Alzheimer's disease, and others. Most research does not demonstrate that using folic acid supplements will prevent these illnesses.

A supplement must be pretty impressive for me to confidently recommend it, which is why my list of recommended supplements is not very long. You may already take various supplements or plan to do so. Before you do, I encourage you to know why you're taking them, to look for scientific evidence to support your choices, and to check for any interactions they have with any other herb or medication you take. Don't part with your money before you thoroughly check things out.

A FEW QUESTIONS

Q: Where can I find information about possible drug interactions with the supplements I take?

A: Your pharmacist is the best professional resource for this information. You can also check for interactions online using one of the helpful resources provided by Medscape at http://reference.medscape.com/drug-interactionchecker, by WebMD at http://www.webmd.com/interaction-checker, or by Healthline at http://www.healthline.com/druginteractions.

Q: What about the popular supplements recommended for brain health?

A: Supplements including Prevagen, Focus Factor, and Alpha Brain have recently gained a tremendous following based on very clever marketing and big promises. As of this writing, class-action lawsuits and Food and Drug Administration investigations are ongoing regarding some of these products. Some serious side effects, including seizures and stroke-like symptoms, have been reported with their use. I can't find any good-quality research demonstrating either the safety or effectiveness of these products. Of course you want a clearer mind and better memory, but until we have better proof, these supplements aren't the answer.

Section 4

MENTAL AND EMOTIONAL HEALTH

Chapter 18

YOUR MIND OR YOUR BODY—WHICH IS IT?

HAVE YOU EVER faced a morning like this? Last night, one of your girlfriends called, upset about a stressful weekend with her in-laws. You talked for over an hour. You were glad to help your friend, but you still had work to complete. You got to bed late and had trouble sleeping. This morning your son was anxious over a test he had coming up and needed some extra encouragement. You missed breakfast. A rainstorm made traffic heavier than usual, and you got to work late. You were already frazzled by the time your boss told you of an emergency project she needed you to handle. Now your heart's racing, your mind is having trouble focusing, your headache won't stop, and your hot flashes make you feel like undressing in front of everyone.

Is your lack of sleep or lack of breakfast making you irritable? Is the extra load at work making your hot flashes worse, or are your hot flashes making you more stressed? Is your worry about your friend and your son creating your headache, or is it due to being late to work?

If you think about it, you already know that your physical health affects your mind and emotions, and vice versa. Just remember the knot you have in your stomach and the trouble you have sleeping after a fight with your husband. Often it's difficult to determine where one part of us ends and another begins. You can't separate what's going on in your physical body from what's going on in your mind any more than you can separate the flour, sugar, eggs, and salt from a loaf of bread. That's the way you're made. And it's a good thing.

Understanding some of the ways in which your mind and your body affect each other can help you take charge of things that are in your control. You'll see how taking care of your physical health will improve your thinking and your emotions, and how developing good mental habits will improve your physical well-being.

Is your body making your mind stressed? Or is your mind making your body sick? It's probably all of the above—and that provides you with many opportunities to take action that can improve your health in many ways.

What Your Body Does to Your Mind

Imagine your brain as a supercomputer filled with microprocessors, memory chips, a keyboard, a display screen, software programs, various connectors, a battery, a power source, and more. Artificial intelligence can replicate and even magnify some aspects of this human dimension. Your brain contains somewhere around 100 billion neurons connected by perhaps 100 trillion synapses. Each neuron functions similar to a microprocessor, taking in data and sending out signals both electrically and chemically. All these neurons are integrated in a mind-boggling way. And artificial intelligence can't come close to replicating the integration dimension of the human brain.

If your brain is like a supercomputer, your mind is like the work products of that computer: files, pictures, videos, databases, documents, spreadsheets, music, and more. The incoming data is processed through your brain, and out comes a creative product in the form of thoughts, emotions, memories, decisions, values, meaning, and more.

It should be obvious that if you disrupt the power supply, install a faulty microprocessor, or run a corrupt software program, you won't get the results you want from your computer. As a high school student, I learned computer programming using the old eighty-column keypunch cards. (I'm really dating myself now!) One wrong or torn hole and the computer would spit out the entire program. We were taught GIGO—garbage in, garbage out.

Your mind can't produce the output of creativity, joy, insight, love, or any other good thing without good input. The nutrients and oxygen in your bloodstream, the substances produced by all your other body organs, the nerve signals that enter your brain from your body, and the outside input you allow through your senses all affect the thoughts and emotions your mind transmits.

Physical illness may function as a computer virus, disrupting your mental health. Mood disorders, such as depression, are much more common among those with medical illnesses.[1] Numerous studies document the mental-health impact of heart disease, cancer, diabetes, back pain, and other illnesses. It's not that hard to understand why that may be:

+ The illness may affect your brain directly, such as atherosclerosis, which limits blood flow to your brain.

+ Your body devotes energy to coping with the illness, leaving less energy for creativity and joy.

+ Your brain may be affected by toxins or altered nutrients in your bloodstream from less-than-ideal organ functioning elsewhere in your body. (This is especially true for people with diabetes, liver problems, or kidney disease.)

+ You may not be able to sleep or exercise normally, lessening the positive impact those activities would have on your mental health.

+ Social isolation or financial concerns related to your illness add to your anxiety and the difficulty you have coping.

Physical pain is especially wearing on mental health. Chronic pain is almost always accompanied by chronic fatigue. Your nervous system has only so much energy available, and it takes a great amount of that energy to process chronic pain. Pain makes your anxiety and depression worse, and the anxiety and depression increase your pain. Chronic pain can become its own illness with a whole host of complications.[2] Few people recover from chronic pain without addressing both the physical and mental aspects of their illness.

From a more positive standpoint, many elements of your physical lifestyle are within your control, and they can positively impact your mental health. For instance:

+ **Physical exercise improves your psychological well-being.**[3] Moving your body is good for your heart and blood vessels, but it's also good for your mind. Simply standing up and moving around can improve your mental functioning. The flow of oxygen-rich blood to your brain increases with exercise, and you know about the feel-good endorphins released with moderate or intense physical exercise. Many studies demonstrate the benefits of physical exercise on anxiety, depression, stress, and other dimensions of mental health.

+ **What you eat impacts your thinking.** You've probably heard of the studies demonstrating that children who eat breakfast do better in school, both academically and behaviorally. What about your late-morning or late-afternoon desire for a snack? Processed foods, especially refined carbs, provide a quick surge in blood sugar followed by a crash—and a desire for more carbs. Protein and unprocessed carbs, such as whole grains, provide fuel for your brain that has staying power. Staying hydrated with plenty of water is also important to keep the blood flow to your brain at its best.

+ **How well you sleep affects your mental functioning.** Chronic lack of sleep can make many people depressed, anxious, and stressed. I'm personally vulnerable here; after a night with little sleep, I can struggle to maintain a positive outlook and pleasant emotions. A ten-minute power nap can significantly improve cognitive functioning.[4] Practicing good sleep habits will help you think better and feel happier.

Yes, your lack of sleep, lack of breakfast, and hot flashes make your brain less able to handle the extra stress you face today. Grabbing a nap, a quick walk, or a nutritional snack may help you feel a lot better. But just as many arrows point in the other direction, too, as what's going on in your mind also affects your body.

WHAT YOUR MIND DOES TO YOUR BODY

Thoughts, feelings, memories, decisions, and all the other aspects of what's going on in your mind certainly affect how you feel mentally. But it doesn't stop there. The mental processes of your conscious and unconscious mind produce electrical signals that travel through nerves to all the other parts of your body. And those mental processes also produce substances that enter your bloodstream: hormones, neurotransmitters, and more. It's not that hard to understand how what's going on in your mind can affect your physical health in many ways.

Stress, anxiety, depression, or any other troublesome mental state can result in any number of physical symptoms, even if you're not completely aware of the connection. One study demonstrated that nearly one-third of patients seeing a general medical doctor for physical complaints had sufficient psychological symptoms to be diagnosed with an anxiety disorder, depression, or other mental illness.[5] Your mind really can make you ill.

Scientists regularly discover new ways our mental state affects our physical health. Here are a few of those connections:

+ **Stress can lead to heart disease.** People with a Type D personality (distressed, irritable, and anxious) are three times more likely to develop and/or die from heart disease.[6] Both general psychological distress and specific traits, including depression, anxiety, anger, and post-traumatic stress, are harmful to one's cardiovascular system.

+ **One's response to stress may affect one's risk of cancer.** This area is controversial, and no definitive research proves that stress causes cancer or hastens its progression. However, a lot of research demonstrates that psychological stress affects various aspects of the immune system. A number of scientists believe that those effects prevent your immune system from fighting cancer as effectively. Even if stress is a minor factor in cancer, it's one of the factors we have more control over than some others and is worth taking seriously.

+ **A sense of purpose leads to longer life.** Older individuals with a strong sense of purpose in life live longer, according to many studies. Specifically, a sense of purpose is associated with a decreased risk of developing Alzheimer's disease.[7] Numerous studies show the positive impact of finding meaning in life and looking forward with specific goals and intentions.

+ **Abuse impacts physical health.** Childhood physical or sexual abuse has long-term consequences for physical health, not to mention the psychological impact. Many studies demonstrate the increased risk of pelvic pain, gastrointestinal symptoms, and other general health problems among adult survivors of childhood sexual abuse.[8] Physical and emotional abuse and neglect are also associated with a range of health issues in adulthood.[9] If you've been a victim of abuse, you know how the physical and mental impact of abuse can affect you for many, many years.

It really isn't all in your head. It may start there, but the impact is very physical. Your body gets the fallout from negative thoughts and feelings, and it also receives the benefits of positive thoughts and feelings.

For women of faith, this can sometimes become a challenging area. Some proponents of positive

Health Tip

Your thoughts are powerful, but they're not all-powerful. Give your thoughts the weight they deserve—no more and no less.

thinking make pronouncements that sound like "Mind over matter," promising that you can change your circumstances, including your physical health, by deciding what to think about. Conversely, others focus on the type of prayer that begs God to do something while taking little action for oneself.

The healthiest way to look at this is with a "both-and" approach. Your thoughts are powerful, but they're not all-powerful. How you handle stress, what you choose to focus your mind on, and how you manage your emotions do affect your physical health. But so do your genetic background, your environment, your physical lifestyle, your relationships, and even your spiritual vitality. Don't give your thoughts any more—or any less—weight than they deserve. You may not be able to prevent a negative thought or emotion from entering your mind, but you can choose whether or not to focus on it.

Our physical bodies and our physical world place some limitations on our lives here and now. But we almost always give those limitations much more credit than they deserve. One of the areas you *do* have control over is what enters your mind and what you do with that input.

THREE WAYS TO PRACTICE
GOOD MENTAL HEALTH

I remember when I learned I was responsible for my own happiness. What a revelation! You can choose what to think about. You can choose whether you will let your emotions control you or whether you will control your emotions by using them as information and tools. You can choose whether to automatically react to whatever is going on around you, or you can choose to consciously decide how you will respond. You can choose to believe every negative message that enters your brain or challenge that negativity with conscious positive input. Those are only a few of the aspects of mental health that are within your power to control.

Jennifer lost more than sixty-five pounds in six months. She totally changed her eating pattern and her exercise habits and is thrilled with the many positive changes this has brought to her life. "People say it's a lifestyle change, but that's not it," she told me. Pointing to her forehead, she said, "It's all about changing things up here!" She would never have lost the weight without moving her body more and choosing healthier food, but it all started with changing her thinking.

She stopped seeing her body as an enemy to hate, focused on the things in her life that she could change, and got the help she needed. The change on the inside resulted in changes on the outside. (And after all, isn't that the way God works with all of us?)

Practicing good mental health habits isn't a guarantee of perfect happiness any more than eating right guarantees that you'll live to be one hundred. Life happens. But you'll absolutely be healthier, happier, and more successful in every area of your life if you take care of your thinking.

We don't often think about thinking. Thoughts come to us from any number of places. Something a parent or other authority figure said many years ago may still hang around in your mind. You learned ways of thinking, feeling, and responding in part by watching others and in part from the decisions you made yourself. You succeeded at some things and failed at others, and those experiences stick with you as both good and bad memories. Perhaps thousands of messages are presented to your mind every day.

Think of the messages you heard or saw yesterday. Think of the TV programs and commercials you watched, the e-mails and social media postings you noticed, the messages you saw on the covers of magazines at the checkout counter of the store, the books or magazines or websites you read, and the things friends, family, and work associates said to you. How many of those messages were negative?

Here's what some of those messages might sound like as you rehearse them in your mind:

+ You're not young enough anymore.
+ You're not pretty enough anymore.
+ You're too fat (or sick or skinny) to be happy.
+ You'll never catch up; there's too much to do.
+ Other people have happier, easier, and more interesting lives than you do.
+ If you could only find a boyfriend or get married, you'd be happy.
+ Your husband doesn't do as much for you as other husbands do for their wives.
+ Spending money on things will make you happy.
+ There's a quick fix—a pill or a program—that will take care of any problem you have.

+ Something bad could happen at any time.
+ Being famous or rich would solve all your problems.
+ Your family is too needy; you aren't enough for them.
+ Going somewhere new or doing something new will make you happy.
+ Other marriages don't have as many problems as yours does.
+ Other people's children are smarter, more successful, and don't cause problems.
+ Problems should be fixed in an hour (or two at the most).
+ Maybe in a few years you can be happy; just don't hope for too much.
+ All those good things are only for other people.
+ It's no use trying; you might as well give up.
+ Who you are isn't good enough; you have to do something more.
+ Your job is to take care of other people.
+ All your trying will never make things better or good enough.

Makes you tired just reading it!

When you park on those negative thoughts, they create negative feelings. And all that nervous and chemical energy coming from a brain that's feeling down travels to the rest of your body. Aches and pains, difficulty sleeping, fatigue, heart palpitations, gastrointestinal upset, headaches, feeling downright miserable—is it any wonder your body gets all kinds of fallout from that internal stress? And much of that internal stress is made worse by how you think about it. (Find more information on managing stress in chapter 22.)

You don't have to be a victim to all these negative messages and the negative thoughts they bring. This is an important area where you can take charge of your own health. And here are three steps that will help you do just that.

1. *Control the input your mind receives.* Most of us don't discriminate thoughtfully enough about the quality of nourishment we feed our mind. Your physical lifestyle makes a difference here. (Remember how a missed breakfast or lack of sleep can affect your thinking?) At

least as important are the media messages you allow into your mind and the people you choose to spend time with. Do you really need to watch all that news in the evening if it makes you anxious? Are the movies, TV programs, or music you consume, the Internet places you visit, or the books you read providing uplifting input? Do the people you spend time with bring you down or encourage you? You have a choice to consume mental junk food or to give your mind nourishment that supports peace, clarity, and joy.

> **Health Tip**
>
> *Your mind needs food too. Are you feeding it junk food or high-quality nourishment?*

2. *Choose your thoughts.* Put up a mental stop sign. When you're frustrated, tired, worried, sad, stressed, or otherwise feeling out of sorts, press pause. Stop everything for a moment. Just doing that may be enough to disrupt the negative cycle going on in your mind. Visualize that mental stop sign. Say *stop* out loud if you need to. Use that moment to remind yourself that you can choose how to respond to any feeling or circumstance. And then do just that. Make a conscious choice about what to do or think next. You have a choice.

3. *Reprogram the computer.* Your mind has the ability to do something truly amazing: it can reprogram itself. It won't happen in a day, and you may need help doing it. But you can develop new ways of thinking, feeling, and responding that can forever change your future. Your feelings are important, but you don't have to allow them to rule you. Over time, choosing different thoughts will result in different feelings. Doing so may not guarantee your body will be healthier, but it's almost certain to have a positive impact.

When Norman Cousins, a political journalist, author, and adjunct professor of medical humanities for the School of Medicine at the University of California, Los Angeles, developed heart disease and a

severe form of arthritis called ankylosing spondylitis, he was told he
had only a short time to live. In his book *Anatomy of an Illness* he
chronicles how choosing to laugh regularly became a critically important part of his recovery.[10] His was one of the first stories demonstrating how powerful the mind can be over our physical health.

Regardless of your current health status, taking responsibility for
your thinking will improve all the other aspects of your life. Your
mind is worth taking care of, and
when your mind becomes ill, it
impacts your well-being in every
way. That, in fact, is the topic of
the next chapter.

> **Dr. Carol Says...**
>
> *"You become like what you
> worship and admire."*

A FEW QUESTIONS

Q: Can you suggest a few criteria for choosing positive mental input?

A: Consider Philippians 4:8 as a guide—think on what is true, noble,
right, pure, and so on. You will become like what you worship and
admire. Read books or watch programs about people who have overcome significant obstacles or have done things you'd like to accomplish. Seek out music or locations in nature that foster peace in your
soul. Spend time with people who are one step further in the journey
than you are, and learn from them. Spend time in prayer and reading
God's Word.

Q: Is it realistic to expect that I can be happy all the time?

A: A mentally healthy woman can experience the full range of human
emotions: joy, hope, pain, sadness, grief, love, excitement, and more.
The Gospels contain many references to Jesus experiencing both positive and negative feelings. Mental health doesn't deny negative reality,
but it does look at that reality and choose how to respond. You can
expect to be resilient and to know times of peace, joy, and love. Those
positive feelings come from inside rather than from external circumstances and are supported by a deep connection with God.

Chapter 19
A WOMAN'S TROUBLED MIND

You have a cold, so you take an over-the-counter decongestant and perhaps some herbal remedy. You get some extra sleep, wash your hands a lot, and stay home from work. In a few days you're back to your normal self.

You're feeling anxious. Your in-laws are coming to visit next weekend, and those visits are always difficult. You ask your husband for extra support and spend an extended lunch with your girlfriend talking through strategies. You plan the weekend so it's as structured as possible. The day after your in-laws leave, you feel relieved.

We don't think it strange when we take steps to help our physical body recover from a temporary illness, and we shouldn't think it any stranger when we need to take steps to help our mind weather specific challenges. Both your physical body and your emotional self experience times of strength and times of vulnerability. And they both need some tender loving care from time to time.

Your body may also experience a more long-term illness, such as diabetes. You learn all you can about your illness. You see your doctor and perhaps take medication. You check your blood sugar regularly and do other necessary medical tests. You change how you eat and start exercising regularly. You know that following instructions and being responsible for taking care of your body will lessen the chance of complications in the future.

In the same way your mind may develop a long-term illness. Your anxiety, depression, post-traumatic stress disorder, or other illness may not go away in a few days or weeks. You may need to take some of those same steps to take care of your mind—making lifestyle changes, getting help, taking medication when necessary, following instructions, and owning the responsibility for taking care of your mind. These choices will improve everything about your life and lessen the chance of complications in the future.

Dealing with mental illness is what this chapter is all about. Unfortunately many people feel shame or embarrassment when struggling with a mental illness. That need not be so. There's nothing shameful about acknowledging where you hurt and getting

211

appropriate help. Doing so may be the most courageous thing you could ever do. Nothing in this chapter is meant to guarantee that you will automatically feel better if you only try hard enough. But taking charge of your health mentally as well as physically is always helpful.

WHERE MENTAL ILLNESS COMES FROM

It makes sense that something as complicated and wonderful as the human mind would experience illness just as any other system of the human body can. There is plenty of debate among psychiatrists, psychologists, and other mental health experts over how important genetics, life experience, trauma, biochemistry, and other factors are in the development of mental illness. And there's even debate over what constitutes a mental illness. We won't settle all those debates here, but I believe all the above factors are important.

An often-repeated statistic says that one in four adults will experience a mental illness during a given year or during their lifetime, depending on what source you read. It's difficult to determine the original source of that statistic. How true are those numbers? So much depends on definitions and how statistics are applied. The real message is that our minds are vulnerable and can often become ill.

Like with many illnesses, genetics plays a role in mental illness. If one of your parents or grandparents suffered from depression, schizophrenia, bipolar disorder, or any other mental illness, you have a greater likelihood of struggling with a similar illness. That doesn't mean it's inevitable. If your parents had diabetes, you could take steps to avoid the same diagnosis, such as working hard to manage your weight and getting blood tests to screen for diabetes every couple years. Doing that would lessen the chance that you would develop the disease. It's the same with mental illness. If you know you're at risk, taking extra steps to care for your mind may not guarantee you'll never struggle with such an illness, but it will make it less likely.

Few things are better documented in the area of mental health than the frequency with which trauma predisposes someone to mental illness. Childhood sexual, physical, or emotional abuse and neglect; domestic violence; rape; bullying; experiencing a serious natural disaster; violent crime; war—all these are known to result in long-term psychological symptoms and more frequent mental illness. Like a bone that breaks or a respiratory system overrun with a virus, our mind can only handle so much before its normal ways of compensating are overwhelmed. And the same level of stress affects each person differently.

Other things in our environment also affect our mental health. Education, city versus rural living, job stress, culture, and personal relationships all affect our mind. Life experiences can either provide us with mental tools like courage, understanding, flexibility, and love that help our minds respond to challenges with resiliency, or they can stunt our mental and emotional development. The people around us may provide us with encouragement and positive role models, or they may pull us down like sand crabs trying to prevent each other from climbing out of the bucket.

The biochemistry of mental illness is fascinating. When neurotransmitters—those substances carrying signals from one neuron to another—such as serotonin, dopamine, norepinephrine, GABA (gamma-aminobutyric acid), and others are depleted or out of balance, your brain can't function properly. Herbal remedies and prescription medications effec-

Health Tip

What contributes to mental illness?

- *Genetics*
- *Previous trauma*
- *Environment*
- *Biochemistry*
- *Physical illness*

tive in treating mental illness affect these neurotransmitters. But are these changes the cause or the result? Do abnormal levels of these substances cause mental illness, or does the illness result in abnormal levels of one or more neurotransmitters? Both may be somewhat correct.

The causes of mental illness are difficult to define in detail. It's clear that all of the above factors play a role. For many people, there may be several factors involved. Your mother may have had depression. You may have been neglected as a child. Maybe you experienced domestic violence as a young woman. And now you face depression as you approach menopause. It's helpful to understand which factors contributed to your struggle, but knowing that is less important than how you take responsibility for getting better now.

Mental illness comes in many varieties, and we can't discuss all of them here. Two of the most common such illnesses affecting women are depression and anxiety.

DEPRESSION AND ITS COUSINS

You may have seen the television commercials asserting, "Depression hurts." And that's true. The symptoms of classic depression may include feeling sad or hopeless; changes in sleep habits; changes in weight and appetite; loss of interest in normal activities; and feeling irritable, angry, or helpless. When several of these symptoms persist for a period of time and you can't make yourself feel better by just trying, major depression is likely present. Physical symptoms, such as chronic pain or fatigue, are also common.

<table>
<tr><td>

Health Tip

If you're thinking about ending your life, call 1-800-273-TALK or visit www .suicide.org.

</td><td>

Some women struggle with long-term symptoms that don't quite meet the criteria for major depression but are enough to put a continuous damper on their ability to function fully and to enjoy life.

</td></tr>
</table>

Less commonly, periods of depression may alternate with mania—periods of time where one's mind never stops. Women with this bipolar disorder may overspend, sleep very little, act out sexually, and behave recklessly in other ways during such manic episodes.

Sometimes, though not always, major life changes or physical illness may trigger the onset of depression. Marital problems, money problems, loneliness, alcohol or drug abuse, or a history of childhood abuse or domestic violence are common among women with depression.

Depression can be fatal. Sadly too many such individuals have not found enough help and ended their lives with suicide. If you're struggling with depression, you may feel like your problems are overwhelming and permanent. If you are having thoughts about ending your life, you're not alone. There are people who want to help you. If you don't know anywhere else to turn, please call 1-800-273-TALK in the United States or visit www.suicide.org. If you know a friend or loved one who is struggling in this way, get professional help right away. You just might save your loved one's life.

Recovery from depression is possible. While it may take a great deal of energy and a lot of help, there are many people who put depression behind them and lead completely normal lives. Read the section on helping yourself, and take action. Get professional help if you're struggling. You truly can get better.

ANXIETY DISORDERS

Feeling anxious before a major surgery or a public appearance is normal. Danger, uncertainty, facing something new, and performance stress can quicken your heart rate and create a knot in your stomach. Sometimes anxiety can be a good thing. Anxiety may provide the emotional and mental fuel necessary to persevere while making necessary and difficult life changes. In fact, 75 percent of people experiencing prolonged improvement as a result of professional therapy reported that a willingness to experience temporary but uncomfortable anxiety had been important in their process of change.[1]

That being said, an anxiety disorder develops when your response to stress interferes with your ability to function normally, especially when that anxiety is out of proportion to the circumstances involved. Panic attacks, obsessive-compulsive disorder, post-traumatic stress disorder (PTSD), various phobias, and generalized anxiety disorder are recognized psychiatric illnesses. These disorders may become severely disabling, leaving those who are most affected unable to leave home or live a normal life. You may feel completely out of control and helpless.

On her first visit, Michelle told me she had been sexually abused over an extended period of time as a teenager. Now in her thirties, she experienced almost intolerable anxiety over even a simple pelvic exam. By taking several steps, I was able to help Michelle through a minor gynecological surgery she needed. While she still doesn't look forward to pelvic exams (who does?), she has worked through her PTSD enough that she can get the care she needs without feeling traumatized all over again.

Anxiety disorders aren't likely to get better on their own. Getting help early on is likely to prevent your anxiety from becoming increasingly severe. For PTSD in particular, you may think your trauma wasn't severe enough to affect you. But if you're not functioning well, get some help. Recovery from anxiety disorders is possible.

WHO CREATED THESE WOUNDS?

None of us escape this life without encountering some bad stuff. Sometimes that bad stuff happens to us. Perhaps the genetic package you were born with left you vulnerable in some way. Perhaps you didn't get the kind of nurturing upbringing that would have given you an ideal start in life, or perhaps you became the victim of a disaster, crime, or domestic violence. Is what happened to you "bad enough" to still cause you problems? Yes, it is. What happened to you is less than what happened to some and more than what happened to others. Comparing your struggle with that of others isn't useful.

Beyond the wounds that happen to us, we also cause wounds to ourselves. Sometimes we don't know any better, and sometimes we do things that make us vulnerable because we're trying to escape in some way. Sometimes we make choices that we know are unwise or destructive, perhaps in response to bad stuff others have done to us. Sometimes it's hard to know where the wounds that happened to us end and the wounds we cause ourselves begin.

In the end it doesn't matter that much where those wounds came from. There are times when it's nobody's fault at all; stuff just happens. What matters is that you're hurting and you can do something about it. Regardless of what brought you to this point, you can choose to take responsibility for your mental health and well-being now, just as you do your physical health.

And then there's the matter of addiction. Is it a disease? Many health-care providers would say yes. No one wakes up and says, "I think I'll become addicted to cocaine or alcohol or narcotics or methamphetamines today." Some people have a genetic predisposition to addiction, and there are very real biological consequences to substance abuse. One can't get over an addiction simply by wanting to. There are both psychological and physical symptoms associated with an addiction, and many struggling with substance abuse have another mental illness in addition to the addiction. Their addiction may begin as a way of trying to cope with other serious problems.

Treating addiction as a disease offers many benefits. *Thinking* of an addiction as a disease, however, presents some problems. Some people use that definition to excuse themselves or others from taking responsibility for their behavior, and that's not good. Addiction is the perfect example of a problem that affects every area of a person's life: physical, psychological, emotional, financial, relational, and spiritual. Treating only the physical aspects of an addiction will not help a person become well.

You can't change your genetics or your past. But there are countless things you *can* do to help yourself from here on. One of the most challenging aspects of mental illness and/or addiction is the sense that what happens to you is out of your control. But that's just not true. The bucket of challenges you have to carry may be different from someone else's, but you're still in charge. Every action you take on your own behalf makes you stronger, and that includes getting help when you need it. If you're a woman of Christian faith, remember that the gospel message means that because of Jesus, you can begin again.

HELP YOURSELF

If you accept the premise that you're responsible for your mental health, what can you do about it? Here are several important steps you can take to overcome whatever challenges you face, become mentally and emotionally fit, and find enjoyment, meaning, and hope in this life. They are:

+ **Know yourself.** Be honest and thoughtful about where you're strong and where you're vulnerable. Look at your family history and your own history. Tell your story in some way; write it down, or tell a friend or counselor. Pay attention to what makes you feel sad, anxious, or upset versus what makes you feel mentally clear, joyous, and alive.

+ **Consider your physical lifestyle.** Proper sleep, exercise, and a healthy diet have a significant impact on brain function. A rested, properly nourished mind is so much happier and clearer. If you're not feeling well, survey your lifestyle carefully for things you may need to improve. If you're emotionally vulnerable in some way, you may need to take extra precautions here.

+ **Choose your thoughts.** Choosing to think positive thoughts is not a cure-all, but it's much more possible than many people imagine. Ask a friend to remind you of the good things in your life when you're feeling down and to question you when you make negative statements. Write down positive things to think about, and keep the list where you can look at it regularly. Practice putting up a mental stop sign when you begin to feel upset. These positive mental habits take time to develop but are one important factor in good mental health.

+ **Pay attention to your environment.** Your mental diet makes a big difference in your thinking. Choose music, TV programs, books, magazines, and Internet sites that demonstrate the feelings, thoughts, and values you want to have. Spend time with people who build you up, encourage you,

and demonstrate what a healthy mental and emotional life is
like. Engage in spiritually nurturing activities such as prayer
or attending church services.

+ **Consider supplements.** If you're not eating a super-healthy diet,
consider a phytonutrient supplement—not because there's proof
it helps with mental health but because it's safe, and subtle
nutritional deficiencies may affect some people with mental
health issues. Consider St. John's wort if you're struggling with
depression. Consider chamomile if you're struggling with anxiety. Melatonin may help if you have trouble sleeping.

+ **Do something productive.** One of the best ways to get away
from negative emotions is to look outside yourself. The world
is not all about you. Find someone else who needs help, and
find a way to make their life better. Do something relaxing
and creative, such as making music, painting, or gardening.
Join a Bible study or community action group. Do something
to give of yourself to the world.

You can make a tremendous improvement in your mental health
by taking action in a number of these areas. If you're not functioning
at your best, look over this list and see if there are any changes you
can make. Make a serious attempt to work things out for a few weeks.
Some people are able to manage significant emotional challenges by
taking these steps on their own.

However, sometimes you need a professional. Let's turn to that
possibility next.

HOW TO CHOOSE A MENTAL
HEALTH PROFESSIONAL

If you've tried to get better on your own and nothing improves, or if
you feel unable to help yourself, it's time to get serious about finding
help. Several professions provide special training and experience in
helping people with mental health challenges. Some of them are:

+ **Licensed marriage and family therapist.** Best skilled in
addressing problems in relationships.

- **Professional counselor.** Best skilled in helping individuals find constructive ways to cope with life challenges. May have one of several degrees.
- **Addiction counselor.** Best skilled in helping those struggling with addiction find a pathway to living free.
- **Social worker.** Best skilled in helping individuals address the environmental issues affecting their mental health. Some provide excellent personal counseling.
- **Psychologist.** Best skilled in diagnosing abnormalities in mental processes. Some are skilled in helping individuals develop healthier thinking patterns and in providing ongoing therapeutic support.
- **Psychiatrist.** Best skilled in diagnosing and treating brain disorders, including providing and managing medication when needed. These professionals are licensed medical doctors.
- **Pastor.** Best skilled in providing spiritual support. Pastors differ greatly in their training and skills in the counseling area. Some pastors provide valuable insight and faith-based support in many areas.

Before connecting with a mental health professional, think carefully about what help you need. Write down some specific questions. What are you struggling with? How would you like your life to be better?

It's helpful to connect with a professional who has interest and experience in helping people with problems similar to yours. If you have marriage problems, a marriage and family therapist or a pastor with experience in that area may be an excellent choice. If you struggle with serious anxiety or depression, a psychologist or psychiatrist may be most helpful. If you're not sure what kind of help you need, don't be afraid to make an appointment with a professional who seems appealing to you. Ask questions and see if it's a fit. Many people need to check out two, three, or more professionals before they feel comfortable making a commitment to an ongoing therapeutic relationship.

At your initial visit be as clear as you can about the extent of what you see as your challenges. Ask what kind of specific help this professional is able to provide and what they see as a likely outcome of working together. If you're a person of faith, it's appropriate to ask about the faith of the professional you're considering working with if that's important to you. At least be sure they will be able to consider the spiritual aspects of your health and how that relates to the challenges you're facing. Some research has shown that for people with a religious faith, incorporating spirituality into cognitive-behavioral therapy leads to better outcomes.[2]

Sometimes we all need some help. Don't be afraid to ask for it.

A Few Questions

Q: Can a Christian have a mental illness?

A: From a medical standpoint, there's very little difference between how often Christians receive a diagnosis of a mental illness compared with those who don't claim a Christian faith. Spirituality and religion can either be a source of added stress or a source of support for those struggling with mental challenges. (For some scientifically supported and faith-based ways to look at healthy spirituality, see chapter 23.)

Q: What about the claim that mental illness is a sign of demonic oppression?

A: This has long been a debate between the religious and scientific communities. Some people with mental illness have been severely harmed by those trying to offer them deliverance from demonic activity. The Bible does, however, make clear that we have a spiritual enemy who is strong and violent. Spiritual warfare should be considered only in addition to physical and emotional factors. Be as sure as you can that the person you seek this kind of spiritual help from has considerable maturity and wisdom in this area.

Q: What role does medication play in recovery from mental illness?

A: Medication can be overused or underused. The very best use of medication is as a means to minimize your symptoms while you're learning new ways of thinking and behaving that will allow you to function at your best going forward. There are some individuals who need long-term medication to manage their mental health challenges. It's not a sign of weakness to use medication if you aren't coping otherwise. Think of medication as only one important factor in your quest for good mental health.

Chapter 20
HORMONES AND THE MIND

NOT LONG AGO, I received a sad and troubling e-mail from a radio listener. Howard and his wife, Janelle, were devastated when their initial joy at the birth of their second child turned into a nightmare. By the time their baby was two weeks old, Janelle had been started on antidepressants. This was more than the normal "baby blues." She could hardly get out of bed and had thoughts of harming herself and her baby.

The antidepressants helped a little, but Janelle didn't like how they made her feel. A month later, she abruptly stopped them, only to become worse than ever. She began accusing Howard of things he didn't do, and her behavior became increasingly erratic. It seemed as though a constant tornado was wreaking havoc on her marriage, her church relationships, her extended family, and her own health.

Janelle's case is one of the more extreme examples of postpartum psychotic depression. Even when things aren't that extreme, we women have a reputation for blaming things on our hormones. Someone said, "If a woman is upset, hold her and tell her how beautiful she is. If she starts to growl, retreat to a safe distance and throw chocolate." And perhaps there are times you'd prefer the chocolate!

Hormones and mental health are no laughing matter. Some women's mental and emotional makeup is more sensitive to periodic changes in hormones than that of others. What would be only a minor hiccup in life for some becomes an enormous burden for other women.

And yet you're only a victim to your hormones if you choose to be. "I'm just hormonal" is not a valid excuse for bad behavior. Your spouse, friends, children, and coworkers are affected by how you act, and you have no right to make them victims of your bad behavior also. There are many things you can do to regain a sense of control even during the times your hormones feel like your enemy.

PMS

Most women with ovulatory menstrual cycles have at least one symptom of premenstrual syndrome (PMS). Symptoms may be physical, such as bloating, water retention, acne, trouble sleeping, food cravings, backache, headache, muscle aches, or breast pain. Symptoms may also be mental, such as trouble concentrating, irritability, anxiety, mood swings, depression, crying spells, or being easily angered.

No blood test can make a diagnosis of PMS. Remember, it's not the level of any given hormone that triggers the symptoms; it's the changes in those hormones from day to day. We don't know why some women have more severe symptoms than others as a result of these fluctuations. To qualify as PMS or its more severe cousins, the symptoms must only begin after ovulation and resolve once the next menstrual period has started.

Some women have PMS symptoms severe enough to qualify for a medical/psychiatric diagnosis of premenstrual dysphoric disorder (PMDD). The most telling criteria for PMDD is that each month between ovulation and the following menstrual period, you have symptoms severely affecting your ability to function normally. I have cared for two patients who became so dysfunctional that they needed hospital admission because of severe PMDD.

There are several things you can do on your own to lessen symptoms of PMS and PMDD. Limit salt intake; that will lessen fluid retention, bloating, and other physical symptoms. Significantly limit caffeine and alcohol use, especially during the time of the month when you have PMS. And don't smoke. Salt, caffeine, alcohol, and tobacco all make PMS symptoms worse.

Stress and lack of sleep can be significant PMS triggers. Do your best to get around eight hours of sleep each night. Practice healthy ways of managing stress, such as relaxation, keeping a journal, talking with a good friend, or praying. Regular exercise four to five times each week is one of the best ways to control PMS and may eliminate the symptoms entirely for some women.

Certain vitamins and minerals have been associated with improvement in PMS symptoms, especially folic acid, vitamin B6, vitamin E, calcium, and magnesium. Strong scientific data is limited, but I recommend women with PMS consider a general multivitamin supplement and a calcium/magnesium supplement. Evening primrose oil (500 mg three times a day) may also help some women.

Preventing ovulation may improve mild PMS symptoms because much of the monthly hormonal fluctuations are eliminated. Low-dose birth control pills may be helpful for this reason, though they certainly don't help all women. YAZ is the only birth control pill approved for the treatment of PMS, and many women taking it find they feel better all month.

A number of other medical problems may cause symptoms similar to PMS and PMDD. Your doctor will likely also consider such problems as depression, menopause, thyroid dysfunction, anemia, chronic fatigue syndrome, irritable bowel syndrome, and others. Blood tests may be helpful for screening for some of these other illnesses even though the tests can't diagnose PMS and PMDD.

Scientists believe the most likely way PMS and PMDD cause emotional and mental symptoms is via the serotonin system in the brain. Medications such as paroxetine (Paxil), sertraline (Zoloft), or other SSRI antidepressants work on this part of the brain and often significantly improve these symptoms in many women.

In the most severe cases of PMDD, stopping all ovarian hormone production may be lifesaving. (If you don't commit suicide or can stay out of the hospital, it's worth it.) GnRH (gonadotropin-releasing hormone) agonists, such as Lupron Depot, are injectable medications given either monthly or every three months that stop all estrogen/progesterone production. The menopausal side effects may be lessened with daily low-dose estradiol and/or progesterone. A steady level of hormones daily is quite different than the wide monthly swings women have with ovulation. Without any monthly hormone fluctuations, these women can feel like they have their lives back.

In extremely severe cases of PMDD, removing a woman's ovaries will permanently halt the swings in ovarian hormones. I have only done this on one occasion specifically for PMDD, but my patient felt that doing so had truly saved her life.

Treatments for PMS

- *Multivitamin or phytonutrient supplement*
- *Calcium (1,000 mg per day)*
- *Magnesium (200–400 mg per day)*
- *Evening primrose oil (500 mg three times a day)*
- *Avoid alcohol, tobacco, caffeine, and salt*

Postpartum Depression

Having a new baby is a wonderful time in a woman's life. It can also be a very difficult time. Sleep disruption, concern for the new baby, and accompanying changes in relationship dynamics can be very stressful—and all this happens on top of dramatic changes in the hormonal environment in a woman's body.

During pregnancy the placenta produces huge amounts of many hormones, including estrogen and progesterone. When the placenta is delivered, the source of all those hormones is immediately withdrawn. Hormone levels plummet. The high levels of those hormones during pregnancy put a woman's ovaries to sleep, so to speak, and they aren't prepared to immediately begin working again. If a woman chooses to breastfeed (a beautiful and healthy thing to do!), her ovaries are likely to remain quiet for several more months. It may be weeks or months before the ovaries restore a woman's hormone levels to normal.

In response to this dramatic fall in hormone levels, some women develop postpartum depression (PPD). True PPD is much more than fatigue or worry—the so-called baby blues. All new mothers are tired and a little anxious. PPD is different in that the new mother becomes unable to function because of her symptoms. Some women become unable to care for themselves or their baby or have thoughts of harming themselves or their child. In the worst cases, women actually do harm themselves or their baby or develop delusions or other severe psychiatric symptoms.

Women who have experienced certain problems in the past are more likely to experience postpartum depression after having a baby. Previous anxiety or depression, previous PPD or PMDD, experiencing a stressful or traumatic pregnancy or delivery, having limited support at home, being a teen mother, or having other stress, such as financial or family problems, increases your risk of having PPD.

Thankfully more people have become aware of PPD, and there are many resources available now to help women who struggle with this. Most hospitals routinely screen new mothers for PPD, and in some areas, laws mandate such screening. Don't be offended if you're asked questions about this after you've had a baby; your nurse or other health-care personnel is just trying to prevent you and your baby from having problems after you go home. Many hospitals will provide information on social workers, support groups, or other resources to help new mothers who are at risk for PPD.

If you're having thoughts of harming yourself or your baby, please get help immediately. Call 911 or 1-800-273-TALK. Your feelings of being overwhelmed and hopeless can be temporary. Help is available.

If you're struggling but aren't in immediate danger, there are several things you can do to help your symptoms of PPD. Talking with another mom who's had a baby recently will help you find ways to manage many of the common stresses of motherhood. Such peer support has been documented to lessen symptoms of PPD in at-risk mothers.[1]

If you have PPD symptoms that don't get better within a couple weeks, it's time to do something about it. St. John's wort has been useful in many cases of mild to moderate depression and may be useful for PPD as well. Whether or not it's safe to use while breastfeeding is controversial; until better research is available, it's best to avoid potentially putting your baby at risk, although any risk is likely to be small.

Talk with your doctor about your PPD symptoms. Many ob-gyns are aware of the problem and are able to help. Antidepressants are effective for PPD and may be lifesaving. Some women may feel like acknowledging PPD and taking an antidepressant means they are weak or a failure as a mother. That's just not true! Among antidepressants, the safest one to use while breastfeeding is probably Zoloft; little or none of it is detectable in baby's blood. Paxil would be the next choice. Several professional organizations have clearly stated their opinion that using SSRI antidepressants during breastfeeding for symptomatic PPD is appropriate and safe. I believe the benefits of continuing to breastfeed are much greater than the potential minimal or absent risk to the baby of using antidepressants.

Because PPD is triggered by a huge drop in hormone levels, some researchers have tested estradiol skin patches as a treatment. Some women respond very well. This treatment should only be considered once breastfeeding is well established, and it does have its own risks. If estradiol patches are started quickly after delivery, the risk of deep vein thrombosis (DVT, or blood clots in the legs) is increased. If used long-term, it can increase the risk of abnormal growth of the uterine lining (endometrial hyperplasia). But in women who can't use antidepressants, or when antidepressants don't work well, this may be a great option for at least a period of time.

Be sure to get some help if you're struggling with PPD.

Treatments for PPD

- *Peer support*
- *St. John's wort (not while breastfeeding)*
- *SSRI antidepressants (Zoloft is first choice; OK while breastfeeding)*
- *Estradiol skin patches (OK once breastfeeding is established)*

MENOPAUSE BRAIN

Many women complain of feeling a little crazy around the time of menopause—and many of the men who care about them would agree. Women going through menopause have a reputation for being irritable, forgetful, emotional, angry, depressed, or irrational. And you're reading this because you don't want to add to that stereotype.

Hormonal changes aren't the only thing going on in a woman's life during the menopause transition. If you're in the neighborhood of fifty, you might also be dealing with:

- **Teenage children.** Is there anything more stressful than trying to parent teens? Enough said.
- **Aging parents.** They have health needs, an increased need for caregiving, financial pressures, and emotional demands.
- **Your job.** The job market has changed greatly in the last several years, making your job less secure or more demanding.
- **Other health issues.** You may be struggling with your weight, various medications, or physical pain.
- **Relationship issues.** Perhaps you're trying to recover from a divorce or trying to survive an unhappy marriage.
- **Money problems.** Concern over eventual retirement, job insecurity, or other financial pressures becomes heavy.
- **Night sweats and hot flashes.** These physical symptoms may keep you from ever resting well, so of course you're irritable.
- **Aging and body image.** The lie that you're "twenty-nine and counting" won't work any longer. You're too young to be old but too old to be young.

+ **Purpose in life.** Realizing you have a finite number of years left on this planet can lead many women to ask deep and painful questions about life and meaning.

We could go on listing the various pressures midlife can bring. The point is that all of these start bearing down on you at the same time. It's often difficult to sort out which mental and emotional symptoms are related to the hormonal changes of menopause and which are not. It's difficult to find research that documents menopause as a cause of anxiety, depression, or other mental symptoms. Of all psychiatric symptoms, research shows that increased anxiety around menopause is the symptom most likely to be related to the volatile hormone changes.

That said, your hormones are changing, and whether that's the primary cause of what you're feeling or not, it's a significant factor. Even if it's not the cause of your symptoms, the hormonal changes you're experiencing may make dealing with other life stresses that much harder.

Many women going through menopause complain of confusion, fuzzy thinking, or problems with memory. Sometimes this is simply due to your brain having too much to deal with at one time. But a number of studies show that women going through menopause score more poorly on tests of working memory than others do. At least it helps to know you're not the only one feeling forgetful!

Now that we've accepted the fact that menopause brain can be real, what can you do about it? The following steps may be even more important during menopause than during other seasons of life:

+ **Optimize your diet and exercise program.** Your brain needs oxygen, fuel, and a great blood supply. Protein at most meals, lots of fruits and vegetables, plenty of water, and regular exercise may help a lot.
+ **Rule out other medical problems.** Thyroid disorders, diabetes, prediabetes, and other illnesses become more common during these years. Get a medical evaluation.
+ **Learn to manage stress well, including sleep.** As much as you might like to be, you're not superwoman. (Find more on stress management in chapter 22.)
+ **Consider supplements.** St. John's wort, phytonutrient supplements, herbal tea, or evening primrose oil might be helpful. (See chapter 17 for more on some of these.)

Medication has a role in menopause brain. Antidepressants can help with many of the emotional symptoms involved. SSRI antidepressants, such as Zoloft or Paxil, can improve mood, may lessen anxiety, and can decrease hot flashes also. If the decrease in sexual functioning with SSRIs becomes bothersome, other classes of antidepressants may be helpful, though they may not decrease hot flashes as much.

I often get asked whether hormone therapy will help with the depression, anxiety, or fuzzy thinking around menopause. That's a very important question, but it doesn't have a clear answer that fits everyone. The brain has estradiol receptors, so it makes sense that the level of estradiol in your blood would impact brain functioning. I doubt there's any gynecologist caring for perimenopausal or menopausal women who hasn't heard some of them proclaim how miraculously their thinking improved when they began taking estrogen.

Estradiol is not a cure-all for menopause brain, but it clearly seems to help many women. It may directly work on the brain to stabilize mood, lessen anxiety, and improve memory. Those claims are difficult to prove. But even if it doesn't do that directly, estrogen certainly decreases hot flashes, night sweats, and other symptoms. Better sleep and feeling better in general may be enough to improve many of the mental and emotional symptoms accompanying menopause.

If you're struggling with menopause brain, it's appropriate to try estradiol. The same principles and cautions apply here as with the discussion of the physical aspects of menopause in chapter 8. Briefly, estradiol is the identical hormone to what your ovaries were making, it's available in FDA-approved forms, and can be used safely in the majority of women. If you still have your uterus, you'll also need progesterone.

There may be no way to know in advance whether estradiol will help your menopause brain or not. Deciding to try estradiol is not a for-ever decision. It's OK to give it a try for a few weeks and see how you respond. If your mental cloudiness, anxiety, or other symptoms are no better after a couple months, it's appropriate to consider other options.

A VICTIM NO LONGER

"I'm just hormonal" can no longer be an excuse for bad behavior. You may be tempted to let yourself feel like a victim to your hormones, but you're not. Take charge of your own body and mind in this area, just as you do in any other. That may require extra effort during some seasons of your life. You may need some help from time to time, and that's OK.

The way in which you see yourself will make a significant difference in how you weather the hormonal swings each one of us women face. If you see yourself as vulnerable, entitled, needy, or weak, it will be tempting to remain passive. You'll see the hormonal changes you experience as something that happens to you, something to complain about, and something to use as a convenient excuse.

On the other hand, if you see yourself as resilient, taking charge, wise, and responsible, you'll find ways to make the hormone changes you experience work for your benefit. You'll be able to see the positive aspects in any season of your life, focus on the things you can change, and take the steps necessary to keep functioning at your best. You'll see your hormone changes as just one more challenge to exploit rather than something that happens to you.

Other factors may make the emotional impact of hormone changes more difficult to manage. If you wanted a child and were unable to have one, the loss of fertility at menopause may be especially painful. If your husband is not easy to live with, your PMS symptoms may only be magnified. If your job is pressuring you to return quickly after having a child, your PPD may be worse.

It's important to have a both-and approach to all these hormonal difficulties. Facing and honestly dealing with your marriage (or lack thereof), your spiritual life, and your total life circumstances is important. So is optimizing all aspects of your physical lifestyle in

> ### Health Tip
>
> *How do you see yourself— vulnerable, entitled, needy, or weak? Resilient, taking charge, wise, and responsible? How you see yourself will determine much about how hormone changes affect you.*

taking charge of your health. And so is using appropriate hormonal or other medication when necessary. Regular exercise and a chat with your girlfriend may not be enough in themselves, but they are important. And don't expect a pill to fix all your problems.

Yes, hormone changes can affect your thinking, your emotions, and your functioning in many areas. Those changes may mean you need to alter things in your lifestyle or get some professional help at times. But hormones are not your master. You can master them!

A Few Questions

Q: If I had bad PMS or PPD, does that mean menopause will also be difficult?

A: Not necessarily. Some women who struggled with PMS or PPD are very relieved to reach the menopause transition, knowing that the risk of pregnancy and periods is over. I know some women who suffered from severe PMS who had very easy menopause transitions. On the other hand, some women who had anxiety or depression in the past may find those symptoms triggered again with the hormonal changes of menopause.

Q: How long should I try using hormonal medication for my PMS, PPD, or menopause brain before saying it doesn't work?

A: Try it for at least a couple months. If you choose to try oral contraceptives or estradiol for any of these symptoms, the estrogen receptors in your brain respond very quickly. You'll know within a few weeks whether this is a treatment that is likely to help.

Q: Does falling apart with hormone changes mean I'm weak spiritually?

A: No. Being a woman of faith does not eliminate the physical challenges, including hormone changes, that we face. Spiritual issues such as guilt, shame, faith, and hope often feel more acute during periods of hormone changes. However, a strong faith provides many internal and external resources to help you through this and any other life challenge. (We'll cover this more in chapter 23.)

Chapter 21

CONNECT WITH YOUR HUSBAND SEXUALLY

C HELSEA SAT ON the exam table and fought to hold back the tears. "My husband hasn't touched me in years," she began. "He spends every evening in the basement looking at his computer, and I'm so lonely I don't know what to do."

Darla felt angry and frustrated at her inability to provide her husband with the sexual intimacy both of them desired. "It's physically uncomfortable, and I find myself avoiding him," she confessed. "I know that hurts him, but I can't seem to make myself get interested."

Wendy wished sex wasn't a part of marriage at all, saying, "He wants it when he wants it but never responds to me. If I give in, I feel like I'm just something he uses and then puts back on the shelf again."

An inability to get on the same page with one's spouse about sexual intimacy is one of the most common problems women ask me about and one of the deepest causes of pain. He wants you, but you find a reason to say no. You want him, but he can't be bothered. Intercourse is uncomfortable. Or perhaps there's some other elephant in the room: fear of pregnancy, a sexually transmitted infection, unresolved conflict, or something in your past or his past that keeps you from truly being together.

A woman's sexual response is a complicated and delicate thing. She may not be able to adequately respond sexually if she's experiencing physical problems, if there's unfinished business in the relationship, or if she's carrying old baggage. As in every other area of life, her body affects her mind and vice versa. When it comes to sex, those body-mind-soul connections are usually stronger for women than they are for men.

A book on women's health wouldn't be complete without addressing sexual health head on. I invite you to come along for an open conversation about this most vulnerable of topics.

THE PHYSICALITY OF SEX

As important as sex is to our human psyche, our marriage relationships, and the biblical command to "be fruitful and multiply" (Gen.
1:28, NKJV), it's far down the priority list when it comes to the needs
your brain seeks to fulfill. Some of you may have a difficult time
imagining anything in life more important. Others of you may wish
sex wasn't a factor in personal relationships at all. But your brain is
almost always interested first in physical survival, and only once that's
satisfied can it concentrate on intimate connections with others.

Anything that impacts your physical health may affect your interest
in sex and your ability to respond sexually. Some women are much
more sensitive than others to the impact of a healthy diet, physical
exercise, energy level, fatigue, and stress on libido. Physical illness can
put a serious damper on your ability to be intimate. While many
women with chronic illnesses such as diabetes or heart disease have a
satisfactory sex life, the combination of not feeling well, medications,
and perhaps the impact of the illness itself may make sex difficult or
even impossible.

Health Tip
Physical pain is a serious mood killer for women.

Some medications can significantly affect libido. SSRI antidepressants and birth control pills
have a bad reputation on this front.
Many women are able to take these
medications with little or no impact on sexuality. But if you struggle
with libido and are taking antidepressants, ask your doctor about one
that may have less impact on your sex life. And if you're taking birth
control pills, you might try another method of contraception if this is
a big problem for you.

Pain is a huge mood killer for women. If some type of sexual
activity brought you physical pain in the past, your brain will associate pain with intimacy, making it difficult to be interested or become
aroused. The pelvic pain, vaginal irritation, discharge, or itching that
may accompany a pelvic or vaginal infection is enough to make you
avoid sex at all costs. So is the dryness and burning that may occur
after menopause. The pain often associated with endometriosis or
uterine fibroids has put a serious damper on sex for many marriages.

Dyspareunia is the medical term for painful intercourse. If this is
a relatively new problem, treatment of any vaginal or pelvic infection

may turn things around. Long-term and gradually increasing dyspareunia is a common symptom of endometriosis. If this has been an ongoing problem for you, please see a gynecologist and have an evaluation for endometriosis. Dyspareunia, if significant, is enough to warrant a laparoscopy for diagnosis and possible surgical treatment. And sandpaper-like painful intercourse after menopause can be helped with medical treatment.

TREATMENTS FOR PAINFUL INTERCOURSE

If vaginal or pelvic pain interrupts your sexual activities, slow down. Persisting with intercourse when it hurts only creates a stronger aversion to sex in the future. It's worth taking some time to figure out the cause.

Looking at when and how pain occurs during intercourse will help both you and your doctor understand possible causes. Pain that occurs on initial genital contact or with first entry of the penis into the vagina points to something affecting the local mucous membranes or vaginal muscles. An infection with yeast (candida), bacterial vaginosis, or herpes will make the vulvar and vaginal tissues more sensitive and perhaps unable to respond to sexual arousal. Treating any such infection is likely to make intimacy much more pleasant.

The unaroused vagina doesn't have enough elasticity or lubrication to accommodate an erect penis without pain. All that changes dramatically with sexual arousal. During the time it takes for your body to become aroused, lubrication increases and the vagina increases in size, making intercourse possible and hopefully pleasant. Working with your husband to increase the time spent in foreplay might be all that's necessary to eliminate painful sex.

Vulvodynia is a syndrome where the genital tissues respond with pain to stimuli, such as intercourse, even when no other physical abnormality is present. Various causes have been suggested, including an overly sensitive immune system causing inflammation of the nerves in the area. Using lubricants during intercourse may help. Medications including gabapentin, amitriptyline, or local anesthetic gels have been helpful for some women. Pelvic physical therapy targeting the vaginal muscles is becoming more available in many cities and is very helpful.

Pelvic physical therapy is also helpful for vaginismus, where involuntary spasms of the vaginal muscles make intercourse painful or impossible. Some women with vaginismus have experienced painful or unwanted sexual activity in the past. To stop the vicious cycle in your brain of "sex equals pain," you'll need to establish new mental pathways that don't include pain. Restoring a sense of personal control is vital here. Biofeedback with pelvic physical therapy may accomplish this.

Whether or not you see a specialist about your vaginismus, there are exercises you can do on your own. Kegel exercises are a good place to start. Learning to voluntarily contract and relax the muscles at the opening to the vagina restores your conscious control over those muscles. You'll know you're exercising the right muscles when you can stop and start your urine stream at will. Then you can squeeze and release those same muscles multiple times during the day, and no one else ever needs to know.

Once you're confident in your ability to relax those muscles, you can begin gentle vaginal dilation. In the shower, in the tub, or while relaxing alone on your bed, use one fingertip and gently enter the outer portion of your vagina. If it hurts, stop. Use lubricant if you need to. Consciously relax the vaginal muscles while you do this. Each day you can gently stretch those vaginal muscles a little more. Once you are able to insert two or three fingers into your vagina without pain, you may choose to attempt intercourse with your husband again.

Commercial vaginal dilator kits are available if you'd prefer to use something other than your fingers. The key is to go slow, to consciously relax the vaginal muscles, and to not continue past the point at which you feel pain.

When you attempt intercourse again, it's important to keep a sense of control. Many women with vaginismus or any other type of dyspareunia feel best if they start with being on top during intercourse. They can then control how quickly and how deeply penetration occurs while consciously relaxing the vaginal muscles. Your husband would do well, for now, to remain still without pelvic thrusting. It takes a kind and committed husband to work with you through these problems, but many couples are able to restore happy and pain-free intercourse using this process. Once you can enjoy pain-free intercourse this way, feel free to get creative and explore other positions.

Dyspareunia that occurs primarily with deep penetration is usually caused by a different set of conditions. Any pelvic problem including ovarian cysts, uterine fibroids, or pelvic inflammatory disease can cause painful intercourse, but the signature condition causing this type of pain is endometriosis. Even if you have no other symptoms suggesting endometriosis, deep pain with intercourse is reason enough to obtain a thorough gynecologic evaluation. Treatment of endometriosis will often improve this aspect of your life and relationship significantly. (Read more on endometriosis in chapter 3.)

HORMONES AND SEX

Now for the big question: How do hormones impact sex? Certainly your reproductive hormones, including estrogen and progesterone, impact your libido and your ability to respond sexually. But it's not always a simple correlation. Many research studies, for example, show no correlation between estrogen levels and sexual satisfaction.

Conditions related to significant swings in your hormones, such as PMS, postpartum depression, or menopause, can impact your libido. But simply taking hormones may not improve your interest in sex at all. These changes are part of that survival need your brain senses, just as with any other physical illness. And it's similar with a mental illness, such as depression or anxiety. Your brain may not be able to become sexually aroused when you're feeling irritable with PMS or fanning yourself because of menopausal hot flashes.

A woman's sexual interest varies significantly during different life stages. Some of this may be related to stress and some to hormones. A woman's libido tends to peak later in life than a man's does. Many couples enjoy a satisfying and active sex life well into their senior years, though the intensity and frequency may decrease. If everything else is healthy in your relationship and sex is happening less frequently, it may be normal for your stage of life.

Menopause increases vaginal symptoms of dryness, burning, and irritation. If intercourse begins to feel like sandpaper, it's time to consider hormones. The thinning vaginal tissues will regain elasticity, blood supply, and often lubrication with the use of relatively small amounts of local estrogen. Simply engaging in regular intercourse will also help in this regard.

During the time this manuscript was being prepared for publication, the FDA approved the nonhormonal medication Addyi (flibanserin) for use in premenopausal women distressed by low sexual desire. This was a very controversial move, in part because of the limited improvement the medication causes and the large potential for side effects. In studies, approximately 25 percent of women experienced a notable increase in "satisfying sexual events," while others experienced no increase. Addyi must be taken daily, it does not increase sexual arousal or the ability to have orgasms, and drinking while using it can lead to serious complications. It will be interesting to see how women feel about this medication over time.

THE BIG "O"

Here are a few things that are true about women and orgasms:

+ Women can experience orgasm, though it's not the same as a man's orgasm.
+ Some women feel very satisfied sexually without orgasms.
+ Some women struggle to have orgasms for many years and are finally successful.
+ Some women have the capacity, unlike men, to experience multiple orgasms during a single period of sexual activity.

Any of the physical factors mentioned above, such as pain with intercourse, hormonal changes, or physical illness, may affect a woman's ability to experience orgasm, even if they don't prevent her from enjoying other aspects of sexuality. So can relationship conflicts, fatigue, or a host of other life stresses.

If you aren't that worried about not having orgasms, let your husband know. He may feel like a failure if he doesn't help bring you to orgasm regularly. You may feel that it takes too much effort on your part and are satisfied with the other aspects of sexual intimacy. That's OK. Letting your husband know this will remove some of the performance pressure he may feel.

On the other hand, if you strongly desire to experience orgasms, that's OK too. Consciously focus on relaxing. Let your husband know what feels especially stimulating. Experiment with clitoral stimulation—gently. Some women find that breast stimulation at the same time as intercourse increases their arousal and ability to orgasm. Remember that you're in this for the long haul. A healthy marriage will often lead to increasingly satisfying sexual experiences over many years.

THE RELATIONSHIP FACTOR

Sex is all about relationship—or at least it should be. You probably already realize that if you're not communicating well with your husband or if there are unresolved conflicts between you, you're not likely to be interested in sex. Some men feel very differently in this arena. Your husband may pursue sex with you even if you're hardly talking. He may want sex in order to feel connected, while you may need to feel connected in order to feel sexual. Learning to both give and receive in this area will help a lot.

Learning to talk about sex is a challenge for some couples. Just as with parenting or money or in-laws, talking about sex can be a big sore spot. Remember that a healthy sexual relationship doesn't just happen. At a time when you're neither fighting nor feeling sexual, talk together about your sex life. What do you like about your sex life now? What don't you like? Is there something you'd like to try that you've not done previously? What would you change if you could? What might you do in the next week or the next month to improve this aspect of your relationship?

If I ever write a book for men, I'll have plenty to say to them about how to treat a woman and what helps a woman respond sexually. But right now I'm talking to you woman to woman. You have more power in your relationship than you may realize. Instead of complaining about what your husband does or doesn't do, here are a few things you can do on your side of the relationship that are likely to improve not only the sex, but the other aspects of your life together as well:

+ **Learn to demonstrate respect.** The fuel that a man's heart lives on is respect. Speaking words that show respect, honoring his viewpoint on things when possible, and refusing to cut him down in front of others will lead to a happier, closer relationship.[1]

+ **Don't expect him to read your mind.** If your husband is like many men, he wants to make you happy and fix things. Let him know what you need simply and clearly. Give him a chance to make you happy, and give him an opportunity to improve.

+ **Accept him for who he is.** You can't change him; you can only change yourself. He needs unconditional love and acceptance just as you do. Are you constantly criticizing or rejecting him? Consider what you can do to demonstrate kindness, true caring, and extravagant love. Focus on what you can give rather than on what you can get.

+ **Don't accept abuse.** You can't control his behavior, but you can choose how you respond to it. You can state clearly what is and isn't OK with you. You can talk to someone, such as a therapist, counselor, or pastor, if things are out of control. You can leave temporarily or permanently. You can pray and keep on praying.

Any bad relationship can become good if both partners want to make it work. Any good relationship can become better. If your relationship needs work, do something about it. Get some help if you need to. Don't try to change him. Do what you can yourself, and he may come along as well.

THE MENTAL FACTOR

Sex really does begin in the mind. God designed sex to be a mutually giving experience between husband and wife. If your own internal tank is empty, you won't have anything to give, sexually or otherwise. One of the best things you can do for your marriage is to take responsibility for getting your own emotional needs met. Some of those your husband may well be able to fill, but there are many he cannot. Expecting any other human being to fulfill every need in your soul is not realistic and potentially dangerous.

> **Health Tip**
>
> *No other human being can fulfill every need in your soul, not even your husband. Learn to take personal responsibility for feeding your heart the nourishment it needs.*

Just as your body does, your heart needs nourishment in the form of stimulation, solitude, intimacy, peace, communication, refreshment, information, perspective, joy, love, meaning, and more. You are responsible for determining what kinds of soul food you need most and then finding or making opportunities to feed yourself. None of us do this perfectly, but you can become better at it. What nourishes you may be a good book, a walk outdoors, a trip to the country, an evening with girlfriends, a concert, or volunteering for a nonprofit organization. Find out what it is for you, and do it—often.

The elephant of past sexual experiences too often enters the marriage bedroom. Sometimes that elephant doesn't show itself until after the wedding, perhaps when some other life stress comes along. Childhood sexual abuse, rape or previous domestic violence, unwise or unhealthy previous sexual partners, sexually transmitted infections, or traumatic mental messages about sex may interfere with your ability to truly connect with your husband now even if he's truly a good man. And he may have his own baggage from the past as well.

If any of these elephants show up in your bedroom, don't ignore them. They won't go away by themselves. Talk about them with your spouse, and enlist his help where possible. Own your own stuff, and take responsibility for getting some help. Trauma therapy has become more effective than ever. The survival of your marriage may be at stake.

Finally, learn the technique of taking a mental step toward your husband. I often hear women complain they just can't get into the mood for sex. Or more often, husbands complain they can't get their wives into the mood. This is where

> ### Health Tip
>
> *Practice the technique of taking a mental step toward your husband, whether you feel like it or not. Your body may well respond.*

you have a much greater choice in the matter than you may realize. Imagine yourself taking a step in the direction of your husband rather than a step in the other direction. Then take some action to follow that up. Give him a long kiss. Tell him thank you. Linger a little longer when he reaches out to touch your hand. Your mental step in his direction may start your internal engines going. Your body may respond. And who knows what kind of excitement may be in store?

THE SPIRITUAL FACTOR

For women of faith, the spiritual issues surrounding sex and sexuality are often enormous. Guilt and shame from the past are heavy burdens to carry. Wondering what kind of sexual activity God can bless may add stress to your relationship. You may feel separated from your husband on a spiritual level. Your head may believe God is good, that He's forgiven you from anything in your past, and that He wants you to enjoy intimacy with your husband, but your heart may have difficulty owning and living out those truths.

I'll state it here openly: I believe God created sex to be ravishingly enjoyed between one man and one woman in marriage. Other uses of sex are too risky and miss the purpose for which God created us.

Perhaps there's no better picture of what God intended the experience between husband and wife to be like than that revealed in Genesis 2:25: "Adam and his wife were both naked, and they felt no shame." They were naked physically, but they were also emotionally and spiritually naked. Adam and Eve experienced no barrier between them or between each of them and God. That's exactly what God wants for you in your marriage—for you to be one flesh with your husband in body, mind, and soul.

In our twenty-first-century world that ideal is not often realized. Divorce, infidelity, violence, anger, addiction, or demons from your past may seem to make that ideal all but impossible. There are few, if any, areas of life where we as women have experienced more pain than in the arena of our sexuality. But that doesn't mean true, healthy intimacy is impossible. In fact, the union of two people who love God and love each other can become a fantastic testament to God's healing power and the very means of experiencing more of His transforming grace.

Wherever you are in terms of intimate relationships, remember that God created you to be intimate with Himself. Our human relationships are but a shadow of the closeness He wants with each one of us. In Christ, you can stand before Him naked and unashamed— physically, emotionally, and spiritually.

For those of you in a good marriage, thank God for it, and believe that your intimacy with your spouse can continue to get even better. Coming ever closer to God will help you come closer to each other.

For those of you in a bad marriage or no marriage at all, know that God is with you even in your loneliness. His love can fill your empty places. He's good at restoring bad marriages. And if you're alone, He may yet have a husband to bring into your life.

Most of all, with Him you're never really alone.

A FEW QUESTIONS

Q: Do women need testosterone?

A: Yes and no. Women's ovaries make small amounts of testosterone, though testosterone production decreases somewhat after menopause. For most women, adding more testosterone will lead to a significant risk of side effects without any improvement in sexual function. If your ovaries have been removed surgically, your body now produces almost no testosterone, and you may have a difficult time with libido. In some such cases, replacing a small amount of testosterone may improve your general sense of well-being and your sexual function.

Q: What if I don't have a husband? What am I supposed to do about my sexuality?

A: That's a big topic and one that deserves its own book. Find healthy ways to fill up your soul. Invest in your relationship with God, and He will provide you with insight, intimacy, and grace that you need. That's too short an answer, and I wish I had more space to address this topic. I lived single and celibate until I got married at age forty-eight. I know it can be difficult. I encourage you to not settle for messages about sexuality from popular media sources. Wrestle with this between you and God.

Chapter 22

MANAGING STRESS WELL

COULD STRESS BE causing this?"

The answer is probably yes. We've been conditioned to consider stress as a possible cause for just about any physical, emotional, relational, or spiritual symptom we experience. And usually that's at least partially correct. Stress impacts the health of every area of our lives, sometimes in extremely negative ways. Our twenty-first-century world has changed the stresses we must deal with, and some would say we have more stress now than ever before.

Is there any woman today who can truly say she's not stressed? If you're reading this, you can probably list any number of things causing you stress right now. But I can also guarantee that you don't want to be completely stress-free. The only people who have no stress at all are dead people!

The problem is not simply the presence or absence of stress. Some kinds of stress are quite beneficial. A top-level athlete or musician has learned how to harness the pressure of competition in order to perform at an extraordinary level. A successful project manager or would-be politician has learned how to use deadlines and goals to accomplish feats the rest of us watch with amazement. Such people choose stress and make it work to their advantage.

Other people may buckle under stress and become ineffective, sick, or paralyzed. And drama queens seem to thrive on manufacturing stress and using it to damage or control others around them. There's a level of stress beyond which any of us would cease to function well, but that level is much higher than you may realize.

Rather than seeking to eliminate stress, let's look at what you can do to manage stress well, and use it in a positive way. (Please note: This chapter assumes you're eating a healthy diet and exercising regularly. You won't be able to handle stress well if you aren't doing those two things first.)

THE BIG PICTURE

The research on stress has continued to expand exponentially in the years since Hans Selye first described what he called the general adaptation syndrome.[1] We now know a great deal about how the human body and mind respond to stress, how the endocrine system and other body systems are involved, and some steps we can take to lessen the impact of stress on our well-being. But there's also much that we still don't know.

For a while, your body's response to stress may actually help you perform better. Realizing the refrigerator is empty may stimulate you to find employment or go shopping. Pushing hard to prepare for an exam or a presentation at work may increase your alertness and efficiency. Your brain responds to the stress by becoming more alert and by sending out both nervous and hormonal signals designed to help your mind and body remedy the situation. Your heart beats faster, you don't feel fatigued as quickly, you may not feel physical pain, and you may become hyperaware of things in your environment. That's all good for a little while.

But if the stress continues too long, those hormonal and nervous signals begin to wear out the very organs they're designed to stimulate. Overworking your brain causes you to eventually lose concentration, have trouble with memory, and make mental mistakes you'd never make otherwise. You become tired, irritable, and emotionally vulnerable. The continued output of cortisol from the adrenal glands can lead to more frequent infections, physical fatigue, generalized pain, and an increased risk of a whole host of diseases possibly including heart disease, arthritis, depression, and more. Too much stress for too long, and your body and mind will truly break down.

That's an incredibly simplistic description of how you respond to stress. Scientists still spend their entire careers researching this area. But having that general understanding will help you understand some of what you may experience when you have high levels of stress for a significant period of time. It also may help explain how some addictions develop.

Two important facts about stress will help you respond better to just about any difficult circumstance. First, your body and mind can develop an amazing ability to handle all kinds of stress if you increase the stress gradually and allow periods of rest along the way.

Your muscles and cardiovascular system respond this way to physical exercise; gradually increasing the intensity of physical exercise strengthens your muscles and heart to function at a level you may never have thought you could. It's the training effect.

The same principle works in your mental and emotional life. Your first day at a new job may be stressful, but not nearly as stressful as if you were suddenly dropped into a CEO position without any preparation. Chaplains, hospice nurses, and grief counselors are around death and dying perhaps daily and develop an ability to manage the emotional weight of those circumstances better than many of the rest of us. The key is to gradually increase the stress and allow time to recover in between periods of stress.

Health Tip

You can handle more stress than you think by:

- *Allowing the stress to increase gradually*
- *Allowing periods of rest between periods of stress*
- *Choosing how you respond to the stress*

The second fact about stress that will help you manage difficult circumstances is how significant your ability to choose your response is in the way you experience stress. Animal experiments show this. Rats in a cage that are exposed to an electric shock will not become quickly overstressed if they are able to press a lever, jump to another cage, or in some other way take action to stop the shock. Other rats that have no ability to control the shocks will become overwhelmed much more quickly.

"But we're not rats," you say. "And I have no control over my stress."

Yes, you do. You have more control than you think. You may not be able to eliminate all the elements causing you stress, but you can choose how to respond to them. Simply recognizing that you have a choice can lessen the stress you feel.

Who would have less control over their serious and prolonged stress than prisoners of war? But not all POWs develop post-traumatic stress disorder, and some who do are able to overcome their symptoms and go on living well. Studying POWs has provided some wonderful insights into what mental factors are important in surviving extreme stress. Even under terrible circumstances, soldiers who chose to be optimistic experienced the best mental health outcomes and positive growth after their harrowing experience.[2]

It's not useful to deny the potential physical, mental, or relational effects of stress. But remember that you can tolerate much more stress than you think—and grow as a result—if you 1) find ways to experience rest and renewal in the middle of your stress and 2) consciously choose the way in which you view your circumstances and how you respond to them. The rest of this chapter is about helping you do those two things.

FIND REST AND RENEWAL

Any player of sports knows that the body needs time to rest before engaging again. Your muscles, your cardiovascular system, and your mind need time to repair themselves. Neglecting adequate rest results in decreased performance and an increased risk of injuries. The same principles come into play with mental or emotional stress. Your mind needs both physical rest and mental rest.

Sleep is, of course, a fundamental way of getting rest, and we'll talk more about that in a moment. But there are also other ways to let your body and mind gain strength for the next round. Your nervous system often responds well to a change of pace. Understanding what elements of your circumstances cause you stress will help you choose the best strategies to recover.

Let's review several options to consider when looking for ways to manage stress better.

Physical exercise

If your stress involves mental work or emotional pressure, a brisk walk in the fresh air or a session at the gym is a useful way to get rid of the stress hormones in your body and invigorate your mind again. The oxygen and endorphins coursing through your blood will help your brain work more efficiently and may allow you to see things from a new perspective.

Time alone

If your stress involves being around people, carving out time alone may be the most important thing you can do. Moms of young children need to guard precious moments when the little ones are asleep or find other mothers with whom they can swap childcare for short periods. If you work around people all day, create opportunities to be alone before or after work.

Time with friends

If your stress involves internal pressure from solo creative work, depression, money problems, or worry, getting around other people can provide a great safety valve. Meet a girlfriend for coffee. Go to a funny movie with a friend. Plan a date night with your husband.

Mindless activity

This doesn't mean vegging in front of the TV for hours on end! I find housecleaning or gardening to be great stress relievers. Try cooking a meal, watching a group of children play, or reading a few jokes. A well-chosen TV show or a time-limited session on Facebook may be OK; just don't allow that to become your primary way of managing stress.

Time in nature

There's nothing much better than God's creation to relieve the pressures we too often feel. Watch a thunderstorm. Take a walk in the rain. Sit by the stream in the park. Listen to the birds in the morning. Look at—really look at—a flower. Remember who made it and that He cares about you too.

Music

Music may well be the language of the soul. Choose music strategically—energetic music to spur on your exercise routine, calming music to back up your creative work, worship music to lose yourself in God's presence. Create a few playlists, and use them.

Special occasions

Every now and then, you need something truly different. Don't forego the vacation you're allowed at work. Find a weekend retreat or spiritual conference to attend. Regularly attending church services can itself be an important part of stress management. Try taking one day each quarter to get away, review your recent life experiences, look to the future, realign your activities, and pray.

Short, frequent breaks for recovery and periodic, longer breaks for renewal and refreshment will improve your success while increasing your resilience in handling stress.

GET SOME SLEEP

Adequate sleep helps you handle stress better. Both your body and your mind need those hours to repair themselves physically and mentally. Regularly losing sleep impairs your judgment, makes you more susceptible to certain illnesses, and leaves you emotionally vulnerable. I seriously wonder at the truthfulness and/or mental health of those who say they need only three or four hours of sleep a night.

If you're experiencing a lot of stress, it may seem difficult to get good sleep. Your mind may ruminate over painful memories, race with anxious thoughts, or try to figure out how to handle a difficult problem. Your body may be tense and sore. You may struggle to sleep just when you need it the most.

A rested mind is much more efficient than one that's tired. Different people work best at different times of the day, but don't fall into the trap of thinking that staying up late to push through an important task when you're exhausted is necessarily a good plan. A task you struggle with for four hours when fatigued may be accomplished in twenty minutes when you're rested. A problem that felt hopeless at midnight may seem much more manageable after a night's sleep.

How can you get yourself to sleep when you're stressed? Here are a few strategies:

+ **Be regular.** Determine how many hours of sleep you truly need, and be regular about getting to bed early enough to get them. Emergencies do happen, but missing sleep should be the exception.

+ **Pay attention to your sleep environment.** A comfortable bed, a cool room, and perhaps some white noise, soft music, or nature sounds may help you sleep better. Turn off the electronics in your bedroom; the smallest LED light may keep some people from sleeping well.

+ **Don't rely on sleep medications.** Instead, try chamomile tea, melatonin, or warm milk. (Yes, if you like it, warm milk can help you get to sleep.) Stay away from alcohol.

+ **Put your troubles on the shelf.** Write down what you need to remember, if necessary. Before going to bed, visualize putting your work, your anxieties, even your physical pain in a box on the shelf. You can pick them back up again tomorrow.

+ **Put your soul to bed.** Instead of watching TV or checking Facebook, try reading a book for a short time. You can also claim God's promises by praying Psalm 4:8: "I will both lie down in peace, and sleep, for You alone, O LORD, make me dwell in safety" (NKJV).

How much sleep do you need? It's a personal thing and may vary during different seasons of your life. Research shows that most adults function best and live longer when they get seven to eight hours of sleep each night.[3]

SLOW DOWN

One large source of stress for many people is feeling as though you have too much to do and too little time in which to do it. Every human being has exactly the same amount of time: 168 hours each week. You can't "find time." Neither can anyone else. You can only become more intentional about how you use the time you have.

Every deadline but one is self-imposed. The only true deadline about which you have no choice is that you must decide before you die where you will spend eternity. Every other time pressure is one you can either accept or decline. Different choices result in different consequences, but you still do have a choice.

Considering what choices you have can be very empowering. Perhaps you feel as though you have too many responsibilities at work to get done during the number of hours allotted. What choices might you have in how you respond? You could rush through your duties and produce lower-quality work. You could ask for a meeting with your supervisor and discuss readjusting your responsibilities or request a part-time assistant. You could research alternative ways to achieve the desired result during the same amount of time. Or you could look for another job. Each choice has consequences, but you do have choices.

Or perhaps you feel overwhelmed with caring for your two young children, cooking and cleaning, trying to keep a part-time job, teaching Sunday school, attending church functions, and trying to be a reasonable wife to your husband without going crazy, not to mention getting any regular exercise or alone time with God. Wow! But again, think of the choices you have. You could trade childcare with another mom a few times each month to give each of you time for necessary shopping or to enjoy a date night with your husband. You could say no to teaching Sunday school this semester. You could hire someone to clean your house a few times a month or strategize with your husband about some tasks he might be able to pick up. You have choices.

There are many tools available to help people who want to manage their time better. Here are few tips to help you get started:

* **Write down the most important goals you have.** Think big-picture items, such as maintaining a strong marriage, regaining your physical health, or developing a skill you need or desire.
* **Notice time.** For a few days, keep a running tally of how you spend your time. Be as specific and detailed as possible.
* **Look at your two lists.** Are the things on which you spend your time helping you get to the goals that are most important to you? You may see some obvious things you can change just from this simple exercise.
* **Ask others.** Check in with your husband or a good friend about whether they see any obvious time-wasters in your life. Don't give their answers any more weight than you believe is warranted, but know this may help you spot some areas where you can improve.
* **Eliminate what's not important.** Does your kitchen really need to be scrubbed that often? Do you need to spend that much time watching TV? (Oh, the things we could accomplish with just one less hour of TV every day!)

Remember, everyone has the same number of hours each week that you do. You get to choose how to spend those 168 hours. And you get to make them count.

QUIT PEOPLE-PLEASING

How much less stress would you have if you were totally unconcerned about what anyone else thought of you? Unless you're a psychopath who truly doesn't care about anyone else, it's likely you

Health Tip

If there's a difficult person in your life, ask yourself:

* *Are they on my side or not?*

* *What would I tell my daughter or best friend to do in this situation?*

worry too much about what "they" think. But then, who are "they," really?

I wasted a lot of emotional energy for many years worrying about what everyone else thought and trying to please them. And I can tell you that it's not a fun way to live. How much better to accept the fact that some people will like you, some people won't like you, and that's OK. Almost everyone is too busy thinking about themselves to be thinking much about you anyway.

Understanding the three primary kinds of people you will encounter during your life will help you know how best to relate to them. They are:

1. **People you can trust.** These people aren't perfect, but you know they're on your side. They care about your best interests. They don't routinely hide things from you, and when they cause you pain, they're willing to work to repair things. They may criticize you, but it's clear they do so only in order to help you become better.

   Treasure your relationship with anyone you can trust. You're blessed indeed if you have a few of these people in your life. Be willing to give of yourself to invest deeply in these relationships.

2. **People who cause harm unintentionally.** These people may cause lots of problems, but they do so by default. They may not have the characteristics of courage, loyalty, truthfulness, or wisdom. They may blame anyone else but themselves for their problems and don't seem to learn from either advice or their own mistakes.

   Protect yourself from these people where necessary. Forgive them generously, but set appropriate boundaries to limit your exposure to the damage they might be able to cause you.

3. **People who are evil.** These people are truly out to get you. They honestly hate you, and they rejoice when you hurt. They actively look for ways to make your life miserable, thwart what you're trying to accomplish, or choose to cause you pain.

You definitely must protect yourself from such
people. Pray for God's protection. Don't fight back,
but stand firm. Limit your interaction, and separate
yourself from them when you can.

Jesus loved everyone, but He didn't get along the same with
everyone. He actively chose whom He would spend His time with.
And you can choose whom you spend time with also.

How do you know which of these three kinds of people a certain
difficult person may be? Don't rely on their words. Instead, look at
their behavior. How do they respond when they are presented with
the truth? How do they respond when they know they have caused
you pain? What would you tell your daughter or best friend to do if
she were in the same situation?

You don't have to have everyone like you. Some people like you.
Some people love you. Those are the people to invest your time and
energy in.

LEARN TO FEED YOURSELF

When you were a child, your parents or caretakers decided when and
what you would eat. Now that you're an adult, you get to choose what
to eat, when, and how much. You can choose healthier food if you
want a healthier body and mind. It's up to you.

Your inner being needs food, too, just as your body does. Your soul
needs nourishment, such as information, stimulation, friendship, perspective, humor, acceptance, intimacy, excitement, rest, encouragement, growth, hope, love, and the experience of worship. No other
human being can provide you with
all those needs, and even if they
could, they can't force your inner
being to receive that nourishment.
(We talked about this in chapter
21 in relation to your marriage.)
Remember that *you* are the one

> **Dr. Carol Says . . .**
>
> *"You're responsible for learning
> to feed yourself mentally,
> emotionally, and spiritually,
> just as you are physically."*

who's hungry. You're responsible for learning to feed yourself mentally,
emotionally, and spiritually, just as you are physically. Your inner
hungers are probably different from anyone else's, and no one else
can determine better than you what you need to do to satisfy them.
Your husband, your family, your friends, and your pastor may help in

many ways, but you're the one who must take responsibility to feed your inner being.

Think of what makes you feel truly alive, and create opportunities to do more of that. It may mean spending time alone to read a good book, getting a manicure and pedicure, enjoying coffee with friends, taking an adventurous weekend with your spouse, going for a walk along the river, creating beautiful art or music, or volunteering for a cause you care about. Few things provide better resilience for handling stress than a soul that's filled up with what matters most to you.

And don't forget to spend time in prayer. God has a way of filling up the empty places in your soul better than anyone else can. Experiencing healthy spirituality is where we'll go next.

A Few Questions

Q: What about supplements for stress management?

A: Your body breaks down easier when under physical, emotional, or other stress. In that light I believe a phytonutrient supplement may be especially helpful, and some research shows they may lessen the impact of stress somewhat. (See chapter 17.) Many other nutritional supplements have been promoted to help you with stress. Those containing B vitamins are some of the most popular. Unfortunately I don't know of any well-designed research showing they are beneficial.

Q: What kind of professionals may be helpful in managing my stress?

A: If you find yourself unable to deal with your stress alone, getting help is a good idea. Some professionals to consider include a nutritionist, a massage therapist, a doctor (to evaluate for any underlying medical conditions), or a professional counselor.

Chapter 23
SPIRITUALITY AND HEALTH

The role of spirituality in health and well-being has been debated ever since the Enlightenment, the intellectual movement popular in seventeenth-century Europe. Some scientists have asserted that faith has no place among people of well-informed intelligence and that religious practices are at best useless and at worst cause serious harm to both physical and mental health. On the other hand, some people of faith have been unwilling to accept scientific explanations for some aspects of their health or have refused to make use of treatments medical science has been able to develop.

Both of these positions are somewhat extreme, though there are certainly individuals and groups who hold to those positions even today. For Christians who believe that God created the world and everything good within it, it's possible to make use of modern scientific knowledge while living out one's faith to its fullest. It doesn't have to be one or the other.

As a physician, I've seen faith provide important benefits to patients going through difficult experiences. I've also seen some aspects of faith unnecessarily create anxiety, heartache, and stress for some individuals. As a believer and ordained Christian minister, I believe we must do a much better job helping people experience the enormous benefits of healthy spirituality while avoiding the harmful aspects of toxic religion. Understanding those differences is what much of this chapter is about.

Being healthy at the intersection of body, mind, and soul is the foundation of who God made us to be, and it's what He continues to work toward in our ongoing transformation. You can't get there by ignoring the impact of spirituality on your health as a whole.

RUN AND PRAY

The story is told of two little girls walking to school one beautiful spring morning. Time passed as they were enjoying the birds and the flowers along the way. Suddenly they realized that soon the bell would ring and they would be marked tardy. Not wanting to get into trouble, the first little girl said to her friend, "Let's kneel down right here and pray."

"No," exclaimed her friend. "Let's run while we pray!"

It's vital for your well-being that you learn to run while you pray. There are some things God won't do for you. He won't take the fork out of your hand if you need to lose some weight. He won't evaporate your credit cards if you need to get out of debt. He won't "beam you up" with some heavenly transponder if you need to get home from work to spend time with your family, and He won't chain you to the bedpost if you need to spend some time in prayer.

Health Tip

When it comes to coping with problems, which style do you use?

- *Self-directing: do it yourself*
- *Deferring: wait for God to do it*
- *Collaborative: God and you actively work together*

Much of this book has focused on helping you know what you can do to become healthier in the physical, mental, and relational realms. Taking responsibility for your health in these areas, however, doesn't guarantee you won't face problems in the future. And trying to do everything on your own ends up wearing you out after a while. There are parts of our lives we can't handle ourselves. Is that where faith fits in? What aspects of spirituality are beneficial to health?

Dr. Kenneth Pargament has spent more than thirty years researching the impact of spirituality on health and well-being. After conducting thousands of interviews, he found that when it comes to faith, people generally fall into one of three categories when they are faced with difficult challenges. One group he described as *self-directing*. They may strongly believe in God, but for all practical purposes they see themselves as responsible for solving their own problems. A second group he called *deferring*. These individuals generally look to God to solve their problems and don't take any significant action to help themselves. A third group he called *collaborative*. These individuals see themselves as actively working together with God to deal with problems. The spirituality of this third group tends to be founded on "an intimate personal interactive relationship with God."[1] In general, research by Dr. Pargament and others has demonstrated that people who face their problems from this collaborative standpoint—working together with God—tend to do better in many ways. They come through various challenges healthier, both mentally and physically, and develop a more resilient spirituality.

That's what learning to run and pray can do for you. You and God are partners in working through the tough stuff, maximizing your well-being, and making the impact He created you to make in this world.

PRAYER AND MEDITATION

Christians have long held that prayer is an important part of one's spiritual life. Talking with God provides insight, peace, courage, comfort, and hope. But does it impact your health? One common conclusion among a majority of studies on spirituality and health in recent years is that what some Christians call centering prayer produces a relaxation response that can promote healing, reduce stress, and improve well-being.

Not all prayer is the same. You know from your own experience that anxious pleading to God when you're in trouble feels very different from expressing gratitude for His goodness or listening quietly for His voice in your soul. The quality of your relationship with God makes a big difference in how prayer affects your mental health. Data from the recent Baylor Religion Survey demonstrated that people who pray out of a secure attachment to God had fewer anxiety symptoms, while those who felt insecure with God had more anxiety after prayer.[2]

Spiritual struggles aren't necessarily a bad thing. We live in a complex world where bad things happen. Traumatic life events can lead to crises of faith that seriously challenge one's sense of meaning in life and relationship with God. Prayer is an important way to work through these struggles. People who successfully navigate these spiritual struggles often come out on the other side with improved physical, psychological, and spiritual health.[3] Spiritual struggles that you resolve over time can lead to positive growth.

That research may be interesting, but what does it mean for you? Perhaps you're wrestling with your relationship with God right now. Perhaps you feel as though you *should* pray, but you seriously don't want to. God seems far away.

Here are a few suggestions for how you can pray when you're in the midst of those spiritual struggles:

+ **Don't confuse prayer with performance.** Prayer has little, if anything, to do with King James English pious phrases said with a super-spiritual-sounding voice with one's eyes closed. Tears, dance, song, silence—all may be just as much forms of prayer in the appropriate circumstances.

+ **Be real with God.** When the "normal" prayers seem empty, you may need to simply let your emotions flood out in God's presence. Frustration, anger, pain, fear, confusion, excitement— who better to understand you than Him?

+ **Choose to listen.** Sometimes you may be too tired or angry to hear much from God right away. Consciously choose to keep coming back into His presence, perhaps after some rest or time. He will speak to you in some way.

+ **Read other prayers.** One of the best ways to express yourself in prayer may be to read one of the psalms. Most of them are prayers, and they express a wide variety of emotions and thoughts. Read through a few, and see if one doesn't express how you feel. Or try some other classic book of prayers.

+ **Know that if it's quick, it's still prayer.** "I'm tired. Goodnight." "I'm stressed. Come with me, please!" "Why?" "God, help me!" Those are very real prayers. What's important is that you direct them to God. His shoulders are big enough to handle it all.

If prayer seems to have become a game of "Can You hear me now?" for you, perhaps for a while you can hold on to the answer many other believers have given. The answer is yes! As with human relationships, your communication with God can be an important part of your ongoing relationship with Him.

YOUR COMMUNITY OF FAITH

It's no surprise that healthy human relationships benefit your health in many ways. This is especially true for those who are part of a community of faith. People who regularly attend religious services are less likely to engage in potentially harmful health practices such as substance abuse or risky sexual behaviors. These healthier lifestyle measures often result in lower risks of such chronic diseases as coronary heart disease, cancer, and Alzheimer's disease. These and other factors, including decreased stress, decreased anxiety, and better social support, lead to an impressive decrease in mortality among those who are more religiously involved.[4]

Social isolation is physically, mentally, and spiritually dangerous. The more social ties one has, the healthier and longer one lives. One of the longest-running studies of spirituality and health followed more than five thousand people for twenty-eight years.[5] Those who attended religious services more frequently had decreased mortality and engaged in fewer unhealthy lifestyle practices. Those same regular attenders also had more stable marriages and tended to increase rather than decrease their social interactions over time.

Seeking healthy spiritual support from clergy or fellow members of a community of faith is one vital component of what Dr. Pargament called *positive religious coping*.[6] From a Christian faith perspective, God didn't design us to be alone. We need the support of others in the body of Christ. Relationships with other believers may sometimes be difficult, but the benefits are many.

People in a community of faith help each other in many ways. Having that sense of community can provide encouragement to grow personally and spiritually, develop healthier lifestyle practices, and give something of yourself to a greater cause. You know you're not alone in facing the challenges life brings. You may be able to provide practical, emotional, and spiritual support to others when they face difficulties and receive that same support yourself when you need it. The community may provide resources that help you address questions of faith, meaning, and purpose.

You undoubtedly won't like everyone in your community of faith. Some people will irritate you or even cause you real harm. God's ideal is for believers to love each other and to support each other when experiencing the positive life transformations that He has in mind for each of us (John 13:34; Heb. 10:24). You probably expect being in a community of faith to be a positive experience, and that may make you more vulnerable when people problems happen. Remember that you have choices about the kinds of people you spend time with, even within your church. And don't be too quick to toss out religious involvement entirely over a few painful experiences or negative people.

Toxic Versus Healthy Spirituality

As beneficial as spirituality is for your health in many ways, some aspects of religion can become downright toxic. Some of these dangers are highlighted when they are taken to extremes by religious cults or individuals using religion to justify their violent or reckless behavior. Counterfeit Christianity has brought serious pain and trauma to people in many ways, and those who have been so harmed hold a special place in my heart.

Toxic spirituality often displays warning signs. Here are a few dangers to be alert for in your own spirituality or in your community of faith:

+ **Command and control.** Healthy and biblically founded authority can become distorted when human beings use religion to exert control over others. Some leaders with powerful and charismatic personalities use religion to extort and manipulate those under their leadership. Some men use these ideas to dominate and exercise violence toward women. Be concerned if you're being told what to think and do rather than being helped to grow in your own understanding and relationship with God.

+ **Rigid perfectionism.** God has a high standard for His children, but He also provides forgiveness, grace, and transformation. Some religious institutions, however, demand an external perfectionism based more on a hierarchy of sins and human rules and regulations than on spiritual growth. Be concerned if your spiritual leaders are using spiritual discipline to control your behavior without helping you know God's grace and experience His power to change your inner being.

+ **Lack of responsibility.** As wonderful as forgiveness is, some people stop there and acknowledge only what Jesus has done to take care of the past without seeking His transformation for the future. This can lead to feeling no responsibility to develop a healthy lifestyle, treat people right, or exert positive effort in any way. As Paul said, "By no means!" (See Romans 6:1–2.) God's grace also provides for your spiritual growth and increasing maturity. Be concerned if your spirituality is based only on a one-time past experience and doesn't lead to positive character development over time.

- **Negative view of God.** What you believe about God significantly impacts your health. People who believe in a punitive God (that is, that God is out to punish you) have a significantly higher rate of various psychiatric problems, including anxiety and paranoia. Those who believe in a benevolent God (that is, that God is out to help you) have lower rates of these problems.[7] Be concerned if your spiritual leaders focus only on God as being vindictive and harsh without helping you know His love as well.

If you've been wounded by toxic spirituality, my heart goes out to you. I encourage you to look for other loving believers in a new setting who can be supportive of you. Healing from such spiritual wounds takes time. It's OK to step back from wherever you were wounded and give yourself the gift of that time, as God does.

HEALING

One of my professors liked to say, "Jesus had only one attitude toward sickness. He's against it!" Jesus never made anyone sick; He always made them well.

Different Christian traditions have varied in their view of divine healing. You may be part of a community of faith where prayer for healing is offered at every service. Or you may be part of a community of faith that believes God rarely, if ever, heals today. But all that theology can become blurred when you or a loved one becomes ill. *Does God heal? Should I pray for healing? What if I pray for healing and I don't get better?*

Sickness can be one of those life events that brings a serious crisis of faith. It can challenge your belief in a good God and lead you to question your relationship with Him. Those very questions may add to the stress of your illness and create their own anxiety. But those questions aren't all bad. For some people, wrestling with these issues has brought them a stronger faith as they find meaning in the journey and experience God as big enough to handle their tough questions.

Physical illness is one of the most important times to "run and pray." Perhaps there are some lifestyle changes you need to make to help yourself get well and be healthier in the future. Perhaps there are some medical interventions you need to take advantage of. It's also always appropriate to pray. Perhaps your prayer will allow you

to see some actions you need to take toward your healing and provide you with the courage to take those actions. Perhaps prayer will
bring God's direct, divine healing power to play and you'll experience
a more dramatic healing. It's important to see yourself as working
together with God in all these ways.

Healing is not necessarily a single event. Our human brokenness involves physical illness, but it also includes so much more. Our
unhealthy thinking, the grudges we hold, the memories we wish we
could forget, the unhealthy or addictive behaviors we engage in, our
broken marriages, the guilt or shame in our souls—all these and more
can trigger illness or make it worse. To be whole we need healing in
all these areas.

One of the wonderful things about God is that He can begin His
healing in our lives in any area. That may be relieving pain through
medical treatment. It may be healing the rift in a broken relationship. It may be providing courage and grace to adjust harmful lifestyle
habits. It may be relief of shame or guilt. It may be a divine touch of
physical healing. It may be using our brokenness to heal and bless
others. The best healing comes when we allow God access into all
the areas of our lives rather than restricting Him to only one or two.

As for me, I'm going to continue doing surgery and prescribing
medication when needed. I'm going to continue helping women make
positive changes in their lifestyle and develop healthier thinking and
better relationships. And I'm going to continue praying both for
wisdom and for God to intervene and heal.

MEANING AND PURPOSE

Viktor Frankl was a professor of neurology and psychiatry at the
University of Vienna Medical School until his death in 1997. He
spent three years in Nazi concentration camps during World War II.
He survived while his family, including his pregnant wife, perished.
In one of his many books, *Man's Search for Meaning*, he described how
critical a sense of purpose was to survival under those desperate circumstances. Those prisoners who lost their sense of purpose tended
to get sick and then die.[8]

Research in recent years has demonstrated that those with a high
sense of purpose in life tend to engage in healthier lifestyle behaviors, develop chronic illnesses less frequently, and experience better

mental health. One exciting study showed that seniors with a greater sense of purpose were significantly less likely to develop Alzheimer's disease in the following years than those without such a sense of purpose.[9] While happiness may be optional, a sense of purpose seems to be necessary for life.

For those of us who are Christian believers, there's no better place to find meaning and purpose in life than in a personal, growing relationship with God. Your small life, as rich as it can be on this earth, is not long enough or big enough in itself to be worth the troubles you experience. But in the larger context of eternity, you can know God created you for a reason. Living each day in light of that knowledge puts all the other challenges we face in a better perspective.

Perhaps the best way to close this chapter and to put "run and pray" into words that you can remember always is with the Serenity Prayer, well known to those attending twelve-step groups and many others: *God, grant me the serenity to accept the things I cannot change, the courage to change the things I can, and the wisdom to know the difference.*

A Few Questions

Q: Can research prove that prayer works?

A: Science has demonstrated repeatedly that spiritual practices, including prayer, tend to improve the mental and physical health of the one praying. Some studies have attempted to show that remote intercessory prayer—praying for the health and healing of someone not present—is effective, but to date these studies have been of poor quality and show inconsistent results. There is no shortage of reports, however, from people who affirm that someone's prayer brought them healing.

Q: Do you believe God heals today?

A: I have both experienced God's healing personally and seen others healed by God's power. I have prayed for people who tell me God healed them as a result of that prayer, and I've prayed for others who experienced no physical improvement. God is not a divine vending machine, where we put in a prayer and get out a healing. I believe what God desires most is our love and allegiance, and He's eager for a relationship with us, whether or not we experience a dramatic physical healing.

Chapter 24

IT'S NEVER TOO LATE

Heather Dorniden loved to run. In 2008 she was competing in the Big Ten Indoor Track and Field Championships for the University of Minnesota as one of four students in the final heat of the women's 600-meter race. Heather, who had already won several track-and-field awards, came out strong and was running well. But with only one lap to go, she tripped and fell, landing hard on her face.[1]

No one would have faulted Heather for getting slowly to her feet and limping off the field. But that's not what she did. In a flash, she was up again and took off running after her competitors. Coming around the back stretch of the track, she seemed to go into overdrive. She passed first one and then another of the other runners, then crossed the finish line in first place, winning the race even after falling along the way.

That will to win served Heather well over and over again. She went on to become a nine-time All-American and continues to run competitively today.

What race are you running? And how badly do you want to win? Most importantly, when you fall, are you going to limp off the field and quit? Or are you going to get right back up and charge forward?

We all love stories about women who overcame big odds. It's encouraging to hear about Bethany Hamilton, whose arm was severed by a shark while surfing at age thirteen and who then returned to surfing professionally and is winning championships still today; or about Condoleezza Rice, who grew up as an only child in the segregated south of Birmingham, Alabama, and who later became the sixty-sixth United States secretary of state and is now a professor at Stanford University. We need heroines to show us that it's not over until it's over and that falling doesn't mean we're down and out.

Those women have nothing on you. Each one had their own set of challenges to overcome, just as you do. They also had the will to get up each time they fell down and get back in the race.

THE POWER OF SMALL CHANGES

You may not be as well today as you would like. Perhaps you feel sick, broke, lonely, tired, angry, miserable, overweight, in pain, desperate, embarrassed, old, or just unhappy. Perhaps you face what appears to be a growing mountain of obstacles: bad genes, unhealthy habits, not much money, chronic illness, a bad attitude, and little social support. You may feel as though you don't have the energy to do anything to change. You may wonder, *Can't somebody just fix me?*

You might wish there were one pill, one therapy session, one supplement, or one prayer that would make everything all right. If you could only find the right doctor, the right nutritionist, the right marriage counselor, or the right pastor, surely they would take care of your problem. Maybe you don't say that, but it's what you would like.

Health Tip
It's the things you do daily right now that will determine how happy or healthy you are tomorrow.

We've been trained in our culture to desire instant gratification. A problem gets fixed in a thirty-minute TV sitcom, or certainly within a two-hour movie. Fast food is so much more convenient. Buying on credit lets you have what you desire right now.

But the good things in life are never instant. If you're not physically healthy, you didn't get that way in a day. And if you *are* physically healthy, you know it's because of your consistent habits over time. A happy marriage or a quality friendship only develops from steady investments made over months or years.

It's easy to overlook the little things you do every day that will determine your future. Here are some small investments that might make a big difference not necessarily tomorrow, but next month, next year, and certainly a few years from now:

+ Fifteen minutes a day reading a good book
+ Walking during a portion of your lunch break
+ Going out to eat one less time each week
+ Substituting one processed food with one more healthy choice
+ Shutting off the TV one day a week or one hour earlier in the evening
+ Practicing a new skill thirty minutes a day, such as writing, music, computer programming, painting, or studying Scripture
+ Sincerely saying "thank you" or "I love you" often

If you read ten pages a day, you'll have read an average of twenty books in one year. Lose just one pound a week, and you'll weigh fifty pounds less by this time next year. Invest weekly in one important relationship, and you'll develop a friend for life. Small actions add up to truly remarkable results.

It's really not that important how many medications you're on today, what you weigh next month, or how much friction there is between you and your husband right now. It's much more important whether you're still smoking next year, how much you weigh in five years, and what kind of relationships you have ten years from now.

If you keep doing what you're doing today, what does your life look like next year? Five years from now? Are you satisfied with that?

If you aren't satisfied with where your life is going, let me encourage you to choose one thing to do differently today. Just one thing. Perhaps you need to call your gynecologist for an appointment. Perhaps you need to begin tracking how you spend your time or schedule an appointment with your husband to talk about something important. Perhaps you need to buy some walking shoes or download the Bible app on your smartphone or tablet and sign up for a reading plan. Do one thing differently today in the direction of the future you want, and the small steps will add up to something much closer to that desirable future than you might imagine.

Small investments over time may not be exciting at first, but like an investment bank account, it becomes exciting when you see the impact of compound interest. Next year, five years from now, or at the end of your life, you'll be able to thoroughly enjoy the results of the multiple small steps you took, such as a healthier body, mature skills and experience, intimate friendships or a strong marriage, and a resilient relationship with God. And those results will mean so much more to you when they come as a result of your own investments than if they had come in one effortless moment.

Getting Back in the Race

Remember Heather Dorniden, who got back up after falling flat on her face and won her race? You can do the same. It may feel like you're down and out, but it's never too late.

It doesn't matter how far down you may have fallen. Even in desperate situations, small changes in a healthier direction make a big difference. I've hinted at a few of them elsewhere in this book, but here are some examples where getting back up clearly improves your future:

+ If you're overweight, losing just one pound takes four pounds of pressure off your knees. Losing ten percent of your body weight decreases your risk for diabetes, improves your cholesterol and blood pressure, and improves your reproductive function.

+ If you're a smoker with lung disease, quitting now will stop further deterioration and may allow significant improvement in lung function. Your blood pressure and heart function will improve. Even after getting lung cancer, if you quit tobacco, you'll live longer.

+ If your family is fragmented, eating together just twice a week will improve communication, lessen the chance your teens will get into trouble, and improve your nutritional health as a bonus.

As Christians, getting back in the race is nothing less than what we're called to do. God has an amazing way of taking our brokenness and transforming it into a means whereby we can bless others. That's the very message of the gospel.

Facing obstacles, looking toward the goal you desire in the future, and getting back in the race is exactly how Jesus accomplished what He did. He kept looking at "the joy set before Him," and by doing so, He "endured the cross, scorning its shame, and sat down at the right hand of the throne of God" (Heb. 12:2). In that future joy He was looking at, He saw you. He saw your current state that may be less than healthy, and He saw you as He knows His grace can allow you to become.

No one reaches their desired future alone. A star athlete has a coach and teammates. An academic genius has a professor and fellow students. A successful

Health Tip

To get to the future you desire:

- *Look at obstacles honestly*
- *Focus on the future you desire*
- *Keep getting back up when you fall down*
- *Ask for and accept help when you need it*

businesswoman has a mentor and professional competitors. We need people who have gone ahead of us to show us the way and fellow travelers to weather the storms with us and share encouragement.

You need two kinds of people to come alongside you as you journey to a healthier and happier future. Look for people who have "been there, done that" and who will share their stories with you. These may be women you know who are living the kind of life you desire. Ask them questions. Watch what they do. Learn from their successes and failures. You can also learn from people you can't directly talk with, women who overcame obstacles similar to yours and have shared their stories through books, media programs, or Internet resources. Professional helpers, such as doctors, counselors, or pastors, also fit into this category as people who can see where you are, guide you in knowing what to do next, and support you through the difficulties.

But you also need another kind of person in your life. You need fellow travelers, other women who are battling obesity or diabetes or chronic pain, other survivors of domestic violence or child abuse or other trauma, other recovering addicts committed to a clean and sober life, or other followers of Jesus who refuse to settle for anything less than the transformed character and meaningful life He promised. Look for a community of people with whom you can join arms with in some way and where you can both give and receive ongoing support.

What kind of future are you looking toward? What kind of joy do you have set before your eyes? Do you want to look and feel strong and healthy in order to accomplish what God has given you to do? Do you want to overcome illness or addiction or shameful aspects of your past? Do you want to close your life on this earth with loving people around you, knowing there are those whose lives are better because you were here? Wherever you are in the race and whether or not you've fallen flat on your face, you can move forward. As long as you're breathing, there's hope that tomorrow can be more like the future you desire than like your past.

Looking Back Without Regrets

Occasionally I'm asked questions like, "Do you think I should try infertility treatment?" or, "This relationship isn't healthy, but what do I do if I'm afraid to leave?" or, "How do I gather the strength and willpower to lose the weight I know I need to lose?" or, "Should I go back to school and go after a new career?"

The present becomes comfortable because it's what we know. Even if our current circumstances are painful and destructive, change almost always feels more stressful for a time before it feels better. And looking at a difficult change from our small and individual perspective can make us question the wisdom of starting out on a challenging journey.

To help get yourself into the right frame of mind, ask yourself what decision you will wish you had made if you look back on your current circumstances from the future. Five years from now, will you be sorry you didn't try for a baby, even if you're not successful? Will you wish you had removed yourself from a violent relationship or tried harder to make a difficult relationship better? Will the effort to change your eating habits or other aspects of your lifestyle have been worth it? Will you regret the risk of starting a new business, learning a new skill, or launching out into something you believe God gave you to do?

None of us knows the future. But we know the One who does. Working together with Him is the best way to become the healthiest, happiest woman you can be in body, mind, and soul.

A FINAL WORD

If you're a younger woman and I had a chance to sit down with you face-to-face, I'd look into your eyes with as much earnestness as I could display and say, "Your choices today will make a difference in your future. You've got time to invest in good health physically, mentally, and spiritually. The life you have tomorrow will be determined by the little things you do every day right now. I urge you to make the investments in your future that will allow you to look back without regrets."

And if you're an older woman and I had a chance to do so, I'd touch your hand or put my arm around you and say, "It's never too late. You may feel as though you've fallen down and the race is almost over. You can't change the past, but you can get up and run again. Others are watching and will gain inspiration from every positive change you make. God will be there, guiding you and cheering you on. And so will I."

Now go, and live well!

Appendix A

INFERTILITY TESTING
AND TREATMENT

INFERTILITY TESTING MAY be tailored to your specific medical situation, but it should generally include at least the following:

+ History and physical exam, focusing on factors that may affect your fertility
+ Blood tests evaluating ovulation and egg health, including tests for FSH and estradiol on cycle day 3 to detect ovarian reserve; for progesterone on cycle day 21 to detect recent ovulation; and for TSH, prolactin, LH, and AMH anytime during the cycle
+ Hysterosalpingogram or sonohysterogram to evaluate the uterine cavity and fallopian tubes
+ Semen analysis

Other common tests may be recommended, depending on your medical symptoms or history, such as:

+ Vaginal ultrasound to evaluate antral follicles (eggs ready to develop in the ovaries), ovarian cysts, endometrial thickness (uterine lining), or uterine fibroids
+ Diagnostic laparoscopy to evaluate for endometriosis, adhesions, or other factors
+ Blood tests for the androgen hormones testosterone and DHEA-S, which is useful if polycystic ovary syndrome (PCOS) or hirsutism (excess hair growth) are present

Several other tests are sometimes recommended by fertility specialists, including a postcoital test, endometrial biopsy, 17-hydroxy progesterone, immune testing, and others. Except in unusual circumstances, these tests are not considered helpful in planning treatment or improving a couple's chance of pregnancy.

Initial testing that evaluates eggs, sperm, and tubes should be completed within one month. Of course, you have the choice to do only some of these tests and wait for results before deciding to complete the rest. The initial tests should be able to give you and your doctor the information necessary to decide on an initial course of treatment.

Before jumping into actual infertility treatment, if you're not ovulating normally, you may consider metformin, used commonly for diabetes but now often used in PCOS. A dosage of 1,500 mg or more daily, divided into two or three doses, may help some women ovulate who were not ovulating on their own. Gastrointestinal side effects are common but usually temporary.

Progesterone levels on CD21 while using metformin will indicate whether or not you're now ovulating. Using metformin daily for two to three months is an easy, inexpensive way to begin, even though only a modest number of women conceive using metformin alone.

THREE LEVELS OF TREATMENT

There are three basic levels of infertility treatment, with lots of variations available at each level. Let's review them now.

Level 1: oral ovulation-induction medication

Clomid or Letrozole is the medication used here. The dose of either medication should be increased each month until you're ovulating normally. Increasing the dose further may increase side effects and won't improve your chance of pregnancy further. Continuing an ovulatory dose for three to six months is appropriate. Most couples who conceive on these medications do so within three to six months.

While taking these medications, you need careful monitoring during each cycle to monitor for the two biggest risks: large ovarian cysts and multiple pregnancy. A typical schedule for a cycle would be:

+ Day 3: baseline pelvic ultrasound by your doctor to rule out ovarian cysts and obtain a prescription
+ Days 3–7: take prescribed dose of Clomid or Letrozole
+ Day 10: begin ovulation predictor kit testing
+ Day 10: begin daily or every-other-day intercourse if using timed intercourse, or begin abstinence if planning intra-uterine insemination
+ Ovulation day: intrauterine insemination (if desired)

+ Day 21 (or one week after ovulation): obtain progesterone level
+ Day 28 (or two weeks after ovulation): take pregnancy test

You can do three to six cycles back to back, or you can take breaks between cycles depending on your stress level, personal schedule, and finances. If you begin your period and want to try again, the schedule restarts with another pelvic ultrasound. Your doctor should review your progesterone level at that time and adjust your dose of medication for this next cycle if you didn't ovulate appropriately last time. I increase a patient's dose of medication if the Day 21 progesterone level is less than 10 ng/mL.

Intrauterine insemination (IUI) is an optional addition to any infertility treatment. On the day of ovulation, a sample of your husband's sperm is "washed" and placed directly inside your uterus using a small, flexible catheter inserted through the cervix. Some women have mild discomfort during the procedure, which is done in your doctor's office. I like to say that an IUI takes care of about half the journey the sperm needs to make, and it can often get more sperm closer to the egg than intercourse alone can. Doing an IUI increases your chance of pregnancy a little, though not dramatically.

Level 2: injectable ovulation-induction medication

Oral medications work by using your brain's own signaling system to coax your ovaries into ovulating. Gonadotropins, given by injection, bypass that system and go directly to the ovaries. If healthy eggs are present, these medications are almost certain to stimulate them to respond, even if oral medications were completely ineffective.

Because these medications bypass your body's own ovulation control mechanisms, it's important to carefully monitor your body's response. Sometimes there's a very fine line between getting one or a few eggs to respond and getting far too many eggs to respond. The risks of multiple pregnancy and ovarian cysts are clearly higher with these medications, but so is the chance for pregnancy.

Your doctor will do several pelvic ultrasounds and follow your blood level of estradiol during the seven to ten days of injections. You'll be shown how to give yourself the daily injections; it's not as hard as it sounds. When the estradiol level and ultrasound show that one or more eggs are mature, the final injection (hCG) stimulates the actual release of the eggs from the ovary. If you wish, an IUI can be done twenty-four to thirty-six hours later. A progesterone level will be done about one week later.

The usual goal of this level 2 treatment is to get two to four eggs to mature and ovulate. That provides an increased chance of pregnancy without overdoing the moderate risk of multiple pregnancy. With careful monitoring, the chance that any pregnancy would be twins should be about 15 percent, and the risk of triplets or more is about 2 to 3 percent. That's still a significant risk, and it's one you'll need to consider when choosing this treatment.

As with level 1, three to six cycles of gonadotropins are reasonable. Most couples who conceive with this level of treatment do so within a few cycles.

Level 3: assisted reproductive technologies (ART)

Sometimes the egg and sperm can't get together on their own, even with all the above treatments. In vitro fertilization (IVF) provides the possibility for pregnancy for many couples who can't get pregnant any other way. If the fallopian tubes are blocked or there's a severe male factor, IVF may be the only option right from the start. And for almost any infertility problem, it's the recommended treatment if three to six cycles of Clomid and/or gonadotropins are unsuccessful.

If you've made it this far, you've probably researched fertility treatments in great detail and know all about IVF. Briefly, this treatment involves taking medications, including gonadotropins, to stimulate the development of several eggs. Once mature, those eggs are removed through the vagina during an outpatient procedure. In the laboratory, your husband's sperm is placed with the mature eggs, and the resulting embryos are observed for three to five days. Sometimes a single sperm is injected into each individual egg using intracytoplasmic sperm injection.

Once the embryo(s) have developed for three to five days, one or more is transferred into the woman's uterus via a small, flexible catheter. Approximately ten days later, it's time for a pregnancy test! Frequently, more embryos are formed than can be transferred during the initial IVF cycle; these can be frozen and transferred at a later time, often with very good success rates.

This brief overview cannot describe all the medications used or the moderate risks involved in going through ART/IVF. The time commitment, stress, and financial pressure involved can be substantial. It's a big decision.

As with any medical treatment, it's important for you to understand costs, risks, and success rates before making any decision about infertility treatment. Ask your doctor to estimate your chance for getting pregnant and delivering a child with any treatment you consider. Also ask about the risks involved, the chance for multiple pregnancy, what your financial costs may be, and what kind of monitoring you will need.

The American Society for Reproductive Medicine provides a lot of patient-friendly information at www.reproductivefacts.org.

Appendix B
QUITTING SMOKING

I
F YOU'VE BEEN smoking for any length of time, quitting may be one of the toughest things you will ever do. And it's also one of the most important things you can do for both your health and your appearance.

Growing up I was often around people who were struggling to quit smoking. Helping people do that was one part of both of my parents' professional responsibilities. I also helped my husband quit after smoking for forty-five years. Yes, it's tough! Nicotine inserts its claws into your brain and doesn't want to let go.

There are many resources to help you quit. If you've tried to quit and failed, or started again, don't give up. It takes the average person seven tries before they quit successfully; it may take you more or less times than that. But keep trying.

Here are a few suggestions to help you take this important step.

+ **Find your big enough *why*.** As with any difficult lifestyle change, remembering your *why* will help you weather the difficult cravings and look forward to the time when you will be tobacco-free. For my husband, it was the desire to remain alive and well long enough to enjoy life together with me.

+ **Find a substitute.** Don't just not smoke; replace tobacco with something. It may be a glass of water, sugarless candy, crunchy snacks, calling a friend, or taking a five-minute walk.

+ **Pour on the liquids.** Drink—water, that is. Drink. And drink some more. Overdo the liquids for at least the first week. That will help flush out the toxins from your body more quickly. The cravings won't go away completely in one week, but many people find that if they can make it past the first week, things start to become easier.

+ **Get some help.** It may be enlisting the support of your spouse, a good friend, or your doctor. Being public with your decision to quit will make you more successful, and you'll have others to help cheer you on through the tough times.

✦ **Remember the benefits.** Your risk for cancer, heart disease, high blood pressure, and all the other bad stuff starts to decrease the day you put down the cigarettes. Keep your goal in mind. Celebrate a day, a week, a month, six months tobacco free.

What about gaining weight? Yes, you may gain some weight during the quitting process. It's OK to deal with one thing at a time. Once you've quit tobacco, you can then make another lifestyle change and lose some weight. Taking it in stages will help you be more successful long-term.

What about aids such as nicotine gum or patches, e-cigarettes, or Chantix? If one of these aids helps you quit, it's definitely worth it. The health risks of these products are mild compared to the continued risks of smoking. Think of it as one step in the process. Once you quit tobacco, you'll need to get serious about quitting these other aids also. But that's likely to be less difficult than quitting tobacco in the first place.

NOTES

Chapter 3—When It's Not Normal, Part 1: Pain

1. Patricia Tjaden and Nancy Thoennes, "Prevalence, Incidence, and Consequences of Violence Against Women: Findings From the National Violence Against Women Survey," November 1998, National Institute of Justice Centers for Disease Control and Prevention, accessed July 21, 2015, https://www.ncjrs.gov/pdffiles/172837.pdf.

2. J. Leserman, "Sexual Abuse History: Prevalence, Health Effects, Mediators, and Psychological Treatment," *Psychosomatic Medicine* 67, no. 6 (November–December 2005): 906–15, accessed November 17, 2015, http://www.ncbi.nlm.nih.gov/pubmed/16314595.

Chapter 4—When It's Not Normal, Part 2: Bleeding

1. D. D. Baird et al., "Association of Physical Activity With Development of Uterine Leiomyoma," *American Journal of Epidemiology* 165, no. 2 (January 15, 2007): 157–63, accessed December 3, 2015, http://www.ncbi.nlm.nih.gov/pubmed/17090618.

Chapter 5—Contraception

1. "FDA Activities," US Food and Drug Administration, September 16, 2015, accessed October 5, 2015, http://www.fda.gov/MedicalDevices/ProductsandMedicalProcedures/ImplantsandProsthetics/EssurePermanentBirthControl/ucm452254.htm.

Chapter 6—Your Healthy Pregnancy

1. A. Soubry et al., "Newborns of Obese Parents Have Altered DNA Methylation Patterns at Imprinted Genes," *International Journal of Obesity* 39, no. 4 (April 2015): 650–57, doi:10.1038/ijo.2013.193.

Chapter 7—All About Infertility

1. Learn more at www.nightlight.org/snowflakes-embryo-donation-adoption/.

2. Ivana Rizzuto, Renee F. Behrens, and Lesley A. Smith, "Risk of Ovarian Cancer in Women Treated with Ovarian Stimulating Drugs for Infertility," Cochrane Database of Systematic Reviews (August 2013), CD008215, doi: 10.1002/14651858.CD008215.pub2.

Chapter 8—When Menopause Begins

1. More than one thousand articles have been published using data from the Women's Health Initiative. You can learn more at www.whi .org. A good summary article is JoAnn E. Manson et al., "Menopausal Hormone Therapy and Health Outcomes During the Intervention and Extended Poststopping Phases of the Women's Health Initiative Randomized Trials," *JAMA* 310, no. 13 (October 2, 2013): 1353–68. doi:10.1001 /jama.2013.278040.

2. F. Farzaneh et al., "The Effect of Oral Evening Primrose Oil on Menopausal Hot Flashes: A Randomized Clinical Trial," *Archives of Gynecology and Obstetrics* 288, no. 5 (November 2013): 1075–79, http://www .medscape.com/medline/abstract/23625331.

3. To learn Kegel exercises, sit on the toilet and begin to urinate. Squeeze your pelvic muscles in order to stop the flow of urine midstream. Those are the muscles you want to strengthen. Squeeze, hold for a few seconds, and release. Your stomach and thigh muscles should not contract. Then you can do this several time during the day (not while urinating). To learn more, see MedlinePlus, "Pelvic Floor Muscle Training Exercises," updated December 2, 2014, accessed July 21, 2015, http://www.nlm.nih .gov/medlineplus/ency/article/003975.htm.

4. B. R. Levy et al., "Longevity Increased by Positive Self-Perceptions of Aging," *Journal of Personality and Social Psychology* 83, no. 2 (August 2002): 261–70, http://www.ncbi.nlm.nih.gov/pubmed/12150226.

Chapter 9—Eat to Live

1. A. H. Mokdad et al., "Actual Causes of Death in the United States, 2000," *JAMA* 291, no. 10 (March 10, 2004): 1238–45, http://www.ncbi .nlm.nih.gov/pubmed/15010446.

2. Q. Yang et al., "Added Sugar Intake and Cardiovascular Diseases Mortality Among US Adults," *JAMA Internal Medicine* 174, no. 4 (April 2014): 516–24. doi:10.1001/jamainternmed.2013.13563.

3. M. Peet, "International Variations in the Outcome of Schizophrenia and the Prevalence of Depression in Relation to National Dietary Practices: An Ecological Analysis," *British Journal of Psychiatry* 184 (May 2004): 404–8.

4. J. W. Anderson et al., "Health Benefits of Dietary Fiber," *Nutrition Reviews* 67, no. 4 (April 2009): 188–205, doi:10.1111/j.1753-4887 .2009.00189.x; Dagfinn Aune et al., "Dietary Fibre, Whole Grains, and Risk of Colorectal Cancer: Systematic Review and Dose-Response Meta-Analysis of Prospective Studies," *British Medical Journal* 2011, no. 343 (November 10, 2011):d6617. doi:10.1136/bmj.d6617.

5. Leo Galland, "Diet and Inflammation," *Nutrition in Clinical Practice* 25, no. 6 (December 2010): 634–40. doi:10.1177/0884533610385703.

6. D. L. Katz and S. Meller, "Can We Say What Diet Is Best for Health?" *Annual Review of Public Health* 35 (2014): 83–103, http://dx.doi.org/10.1146/annurev-publhealth-032013-182351.

7. Ramón Estruch et al., "Primary Prevention of Cardiovascular Disease with a Mediterranean Diet," *New England Journal of Medicine* 368 (April 4, 2013): 1279–90. doi:10.1056/NEJMoa1200303.

8. Learn more about Kathrine Lee at www.ilivethesource.com.

9. Sabine Rohrmann et al., "Meat Consumption and Mortality— Results From the European Prospective Investigation Into Cancer and Nutrition," *BMC Medicine* 11 (2013): 63. doi:10.1186/1741-7015-11-63.

10. N. R. Damasceno et al., "Crossover Study of Diets Enriched With Virgin Olive Oil, Walnuts, or Almonds. Effects on Lipids and Other Cardiovascular Risk Markers," *Nutrition, Metabolism, and Cardiovascular Diseases* 21, suppl. 1 (June 2011): S14–20. doi:10.1016/j.numecd.2010.12.006.

11. Hongyu Wu et al., "Association Between Dietary Whole Grain Intake and Risk of Mortality: Two Large Prospective Studies in US Men and Women," *JAMA Internal Medicine* 175, no. 3 (March 2015): 373–84. doi:10.1001/jamainternmed.2014.6283.

CHAPTER 10—MANAGING YOUR WEIGHT

1. Helen L. Walls et al., "Obesity and Trends in Life Expectancy," *Journal of Obesity* 2012 (2012): 107989. doi:10.1155/2012/107989.

2. J. P. Moriarty et al., "The Effects of Incremental Costs of Smoking and Obesity on Health Care Costs Among Adults: A 7-Year Longitudinal Study," *Journal of Occupational and Environmental Medicine* 54, no. 3 (March 2012): 286–91. doi:10.1097/JOM.0b013e318246f1f4.

3. "The US Weight Loss and Diet Control Market," Marketdata Enterprises, March 1, 2013, accessed July 21, 2015, http://www.marketresearch.com/Marketdata-Enterprises-Inc-v416/Weight-Loss-Diet-Control-7468694/.

4. You can calculate your body mass index on the National Heart, Lung, and Blood Institute's website at http://www.nhlbi.nih.gov/health/educational/lose_wt/BMI/bmicalc.htm.

CHAPTER 11—CANCER PREVENTION FOR WOMEN

1. "Lifetime Risk of Developing or Dying From Cancer," American Cancer Society, last revised October 1, 2014, accessed July 21, 2015, http://www.cancer.org/cancer/cancerbasics/lifetime-probability-of-developing-or-dying-from-cancer.

2. *Cancer Facts and Figures 2014* (Atlanta: American Cancer Society, 2014), 43.

3. Ibid., 53.

4. Ibid., 55.

5. Marcia L. Stefanick et al., "Effects of Conjugated Equine Estrogens on Breast Cancer and Mammography Screening in Postmenopausal Women With Hysterectomy," *JAMA* 295, no. 14 (2006): 1647–57. doi:10.1001/jama.295.14.1647.

6. Katharine A. Dobson Amato et al., "Tobacco Cessation May Improve Lung Cancer Patient Survival," *Journal of Thoracic Oncology* 10, no. 7 (July 2015): 1014–19. doi:10.1097/JTO.0000000000000578.

7. Xiangli Cui et al., "Suppression of DNA Damage in Human Peripheral Blood Lymphocytes by a Juice Concentrate: A Randomized, Double-Blind, Placebo-Controlled Trial," *Molecular Nutrition & Food Research* 56, no. 4 (April 2012): 666–70. doi:10.1002/mnfr.201100496.

Chapter 12—Diseases Older Women Face

1. For several fascinating infographics on causes of death, see David S. Jones, Scott H. Podolsky, and Jeremy A. Greene, "The Burden of Disease and the Changing Task of Medicine," *New England Journal of Medicine* 366 (2012): 2333–38, accessed July 21, 2015, http://www.nejm.org/doi/full/10.1056/NEJMp1113569.

2. Learn more at www.goredforwomen.org.

3. A. K. Chomistek et al., "Healthy Lifestyle in the Primordial Prevention of Cardiovascular Disease Among Young Women," *Journal of the American College of Cardiology* 65, no. 1 (January 6, 2015): 43–51. doi:10.1016/j.jacc.2014.10.024.

4. Statistics in this section were gathered from the Centers for Disease Control and Prevention, available at www.cdc.gov/diabetes.

Chapter 13—Staying Younger Longer

1. "Antiaging Products and Services: The Global Market," BCC Research, August 2013, accessed July 21, 2015, http://www.bccresearch.com/market-research/healthcare/antiaging-products-services-hlc060b.html.

2. Dylan Thomas, *The Poems of Dylan Thomas*, rev. ed. (New York: New Directions, 2003), 239.

3. Becca R. Levy et al., "Association Between Positive Age Stereotypes and Recovery From Disability in Older Persons," *JAMA* 308, no. 19 (November 21, 2012): 1972–73. doi:10.1001/jama.2012.14541.

4. "NIH-Supported Study Finds US Dementia Care Costs as High as $215 Billion in 2010," National Institutes of Health, April 3, 2013, accessed July 21, 2015, http://www.nih.gov/news/health/apr2013/nia-03.htm.

5. Tom C. Russ et al., "Psychological Distress as a Risk Factor for Dementia Death," *Archives of Internal Medicine* 171, no. 20 (2011): 1859. doi:10.1001/archinternmed.2011.521.

6. Patricia A. Boyle et al., "Effect of a Purpose in Life on Risk of Incident Alzheimer Disease and Mild Cognitive Impairment in Community-Dwelling Older Persons," *Archives of General Psychiatry* 67, no. 3 (March 2010): 304–10. doi:10.1001/archgenpsychiatry.2009.208.

7. M. C. Voelkle, "Let Me Guess How Old You Are: Effects of Age, Gender, and Facial Expression on Perceptions of Age," *Psychology and Aging* 27, no. 2 (June 2012): 265–77. doi:10.1037/a0025065.

8. M. Pahor et al., "Effect of Structured Physical Activity on Prevention of Major Mobility Disability in Older Adults: The LIFE Study Randomized Clinical Trial," *JAMA* 311, no. 23 (June 18, 2014): 2387–96. doi:10.1001/jama.2014.5616.

9. Arthur F. Kramer, Kirk I. Erickson, and Stanley J. Colcombe, "Exercise, Cognition, and the Aging Brain," *Journal of Applied Physiology* 101, no. 4 (October 2006): 1237–42. doi:10.1152/japplphysiol.00500.2006.

10. John T. Cacioppo and Stephanie Cacioppo, "Social Relationships and Health: The Toxic Effects of Perceived Social Isolation," *Social and Personality Psychology Compass* 8, no. 2 (February 2014): 58–72. doi:10.1111/spc3.12087.

11. "Wrinkle Creams: Miracle or Mirage?" *Consumer Reports*, September 2011, accessed July 21, 2015, http://www.consumerreports.org/cro/magazine-archive/2011/september/health/wrinkle-creams/overview/index.htm.

CHAPTER 14—VISITING YOUR DOCTOR

1. Erin McCann, "HIPAA Data Breaches Climb 138 Percent," February 6, 2014, *Healthcare IT News*, accessed July 21, 2015, http://www.healthcareitnews.com/news/hipaa-data-breaches-climb-138-percent.

CHAPTER 15—DO YOU REALLY NEED THAT TEST?

1. Learn more at www.uspreventiveservicestaskforce.org.

2. "What Are the Survival Rates for Colorectal Cancer by Stage?" American Cancer Society, last revised August 13, 2015, accessed July 21, 2015, http://www.cancer.org/cancer/colonandrectumcancer/detailedguide/colorectal-cancer-survival-rates.

3. Calculate your risk for experiencing a heart attack in the next ten years by using the tools available at http://www.chd-taskforce.de/coronary_risk_assessment.html and http://cvdrisk.nhlbi.nih.gov/calculator.asp.

Chapter 16—Navigating the Health-Care System

1. "Health Expenditure, Total (% of GDP)," The World Bank, accessed July 21, 2015, http://data.worldbank.org/indicator/SH.XPD.TOTL.ZS.

2. Christina LaMontagne, "NerdWallet Health Finds Medical Bankruptcy Accounts for Majority of Personal Bankruptcies," March 26, 2014, NerdWallet.com, accessed July 21, 2015, http://www.nerdwallet.com/blog/health/2014/03/26/medical-bankruptcy/.

Chapter 17—Evaluating and Using Supplements

1. "NBJ's Global Supplement and Nutrition Industry Report, 2014," *Nutrition Business Journal*, Penton Media, accessed July 21, 2015, http://newhope360.com/site-files/newhope360.com/files/uploads/2014/Global_Report%20summary.pdf.

2. Yu Jin et al., "Systemic Inflammatory Load in Humans Is Suppressed by Consumption of Two Formulations of Dried, Encapsulated Juice Concentrate," *Molecular Nutrition and Food Research* 54, no. 10 (October 2010): 1506–14. doi:10.1002/mnfr.200900579.

3. Meri P. Nantz et al., "Immunity and Antioxidant Capacity in Humans Is Enhanced by Consumption of a Dried, Encapsulated Fruit and Vegetable Juice Concentrate," *Journal of Nutrition* 136, no. 10 (October 2006): 2606–10, http://jn.nutrition.org/content/136/10/2606.full.pdf+html.

4. See Antonio Simone Laganà and Alfonsa Pizzo, "Know Your Enemy: The Rationale of Using Inositol in the Treatment of Polycystic Ovary Syndrome," *Endocrinology and Metabolic Syndrome* 2 (November 2013): e121. doi:10.4172/2161-1017.1000e121.

5. Maurizio Nordio and E. Proietti, "The Combined Therapy With Myo-Inositol and D-Chiro-Inositol Reduces the Risk of Metabolic Disease in PCOS Overweight Patients Compared to Myo-Inositol Supplementation Alone," *European Review for Medical and Pharmacological Sciences* 16, no. 5 (May 2012): 575–81, http://www.researchgate.net/publication/229006272_The_Combined_therapy_with_myo-inositol_and_D-Chiro-inositol_reduces_the_risk_of_metabolic_disease_in_PCOS_overweight_patients_compared_to_myo-inositol_supplementation_alone.

6. J. Mursu et al., "Dietary Supplements and Mortality Rate in Older Women: the Iowa Women's Health Study," *Archives of Internal Medicine* 171, no. 18 (October 10, 2011): 1625–33. doi:10.1001/archinternmed.2011.445.

7. J. M. Gaziano et al., "Multivitamins in the Prevention of Cancer in Men: the Physicians' Health Study II Randomized Controlled Trial," *JAMA* 308, no. 18 (November 14, 2012): 1871–80, http://www.ncbi.nlm.nih.gov/pubmed/23162860/.

8. Shinichi Kuriyama et al., "Green Tea Consumption and Mortality Due to Cardiovascular Disease, Cancer, and All Causes in Japan: the Ohsaki Study," *JAMA* 296, no. 10 (September 13, 2006): 1255–65. doi:10.1001/jama.296.10.1255.

9. Salman K. Bhatti, James H. O'Keefe, and Carl J. Lavie, "Coffee and Tea: Perks for Health and Longevity?" *Current Opinion in Clinical Nutrition and Metabolic Care* 16, no. 6 (November 2013): 688–97. doi:10.1097 /MCO.0b013e328365b9a0.

CHAPTER 18—YOUR MIND OR YOUR BODY—WHICH IS IT?

1. Dwight L. Evans et al., "Mood Disorders in the Medically Ill: Scientific Review and Recommendations," *Biological Psychiatry* 58, no. 3 (August 1, 2005): 175–89, http://dx.doi.org/10.1016/j.biopsych.2005.05.001.

2. Perry G. Fine, "Long-Term Consequences of Chronic Pain: Mounting Evidence for Pain as a Neurological Disease and Parallels With Other Chronic Disease States," *Pain Medicine* 12, no. 7 (July 2011): 996–1004. doi:10.1111/j.1526-4637.2011.01187.x.

3. Peter Hassmén, Nathalie Koivula, and Antti Uutela, "Physical Exercise and Psychological Well-Being: A Population Study in Finland," *Preventive Medicine* 30, no. 1 (January 2000): 17–25. doi:10.1006/pmed .1999.0597.

4. Nicole Lovato and Leon Lack, "The Effects of Napping on Cognitive Functioning," *Progress in Brain Research* 185 (January 2010): 155–66. doi:10.1016/B978-0-444-53702-7.00009-9.

5. Nader Haftgoli et al., "Patients Presenting With Somatic Complaints in General Practice: Depression, Anxiety, and Somatoform Disorders Are Frequent and Associated With Psychosocial Stressors," *BMC Family Practice* 11 (2010): 67. doi:10.1186/1471-2296-11-67.

6. Johan Denollet, Angélique A. Schiffer, and Viola Spek, "A General Propensity to Psychological Distress Affects Cardiovascular Outcomes: Evidence on the Type D (Distressed) Personality Profile," *Circulation: Cardiovascular Quality and Outcomes* 3 (2010): 546–57. doi:10.1161/CIR COUTCOMES.109.934406.

7. Boyle et al., "Effect of a Purpose in Life."

8. Leah Irish, Ihori Kobayashi, and Douglas L. Delahanty, "Long-Term Physical Health Consequences of Childhood Sexual Abuse: A Meta-Analytic Review," *Journal of Pediatric Psychology* 35, no. 5 (2010): 450–61. doi:10.1093/jpepsy/jsp118.

9. Rosana E. Norman et al., "The Long-Term Health Consequences of Child Physical Abuse, Emotional Abuse, and Neglect: A Systematic Review and Meta-Analysis," *PLoS Medicine* 9, no. 11 (November 2012): e1001349. doi:10.1371/journal.pmed.1001349.

10. Norman Cousins, *Anatomy of an Illness: As Perceived by the Patient: Twentieth Anniversary Edition*, (New York, NY: Norton & Company Ltd., 2005).

CHAPTER 19—A WOMAN'S TROUBLED MIND

1. Fred J. Hanna and Martin H. Ritchie, "Seeking the Active Ingredients of Psychotherapeutic Change: Within and Outside the Context of Therapy," *Professional Psychology: Research and Practice* 26, no. 2 (April 1995): 176–83. doi:10.1037/0735-7028.26.2.176.

2. L. Rebecca Propst, "Comparative Efficacy of Religious and Nonreligious Cognitive-Behavioral Therapy for the Treatment of Clinical Depression in Religious Individuals," *Journal of Consulting and Clinical Psychology* 60, no. 1 (February 1992): 94–103. doi:10.1007/BF01173648.

CHAPTER 20—HORMONES AND THE MIND

1. Joni Leger and Nicole Letourneau, "New Mothers and Postpartum Depression: A Narrative Review of Peer Support Intervention Studies," *Health and Social Care in the Community* 23, no. 4 (July 2015), 337–48. doi:10.1111/hsc.12125.

CHAPTER 21—CONNECT WITH YOUR HUSBAND SEXUALLY

1. For a good resource about how important respect is to a man's heart, see Emerson Eggerichs, *Love and Respect: The Love She Most Desires, The Respect He Desperately Needs* (Nashville, TN: Thomas Nelson, 2004).

CHAPTER 22—MANAGING STRESS WELL

1. Hans Selye, "Stress and the General Adaptation Syndrome," *British Medical Journal* 1, no. 4667 (June 1950): 1383–92, http://www.jstor.org /stable/25357371.

2. A. Feder et al., "Posttraumatic Growth in Former Vietnam Prisoners of War," *Psychiatry* 71, no. 4 (Winter 2008): 359–70, http://www .medscape.com/medline/abstract/19152285.

3. Francesco P. Cappuccio et al., "Sleep Duration and All-Cause Mortality: A Systematic Review and Meta-Analysis of Prospective Studies," *Sleep* 33, no. 5 (May 2010): 585–92, http://www.ncbi.nlm.nih.gov/pmc /articles/PMC2864873/?ncid=txtlnkusaolp00000618.

CHAPTER 23—SPIRITUALITY AND HEALTH

1. Kenneth I. Pargament et al., "Religion and the Problem-Solving Process: Three Styles of Coping," *Journal for the Scientific Study of Religion* 27, no. 1 (March 1998): 99, doi:10.2307/1387404.

2. Christopher G. Ellison et al., "Prayer, Attachment to God, and Symptoms of Anxiety-Related Disorders Among US Adults," *Sociology of Religion* 75, no. 2 (Summer 2014): 208–33. doi: 10.1093/socrel/srt079.

3. Kenneth I. Pargament et al., "Religious Coping Methods as Predictors of Psychological, Physical, and Spiritual Outcomes Among Medically Ill Elderly Patients: A Two-Year Longitudinal Study," *Journal of Health Psychology* 9, no. 6 (November 2004): 713–730. doi:10.1177/1359105304045366.

4. Harold G. Koenig, "Religion, Spirituality, and Health: The Research and Clinical Implications," *ISRN Psychiatry* 2012 (2012): 1194–200. doi:10.5402/2012/278730.

5. W. J. Strawbridge et al., "Frequent Attendance at Religious Services and Mortality Over Twenty-Eight Years," *American Journal of Public Health* 87, no. 6 (June 1997): 957–61, http://www.ncbi.nlm.nih.gov/pmc/articles/PMC1380930/.

6. Kenneth I. Pargament et al., "Patterns of Positive and Negative Religious Coping With Major Life Stressors," *Journal for the Scientific Study of Religion* 37, no. 4 (December 1998): 710–24. doi:10.2307/1388152.

7. Nava R. Silton et al., "Beliefs About God and Mental Health Among American Adults," *Journal of Religion and Health* 53, no. 5 (October 2014): 1285–96, http://dx.doi.org/10.1007/s10943-013-9712-3.

8. Viktor Frankl, *Man's Search for Meaning* (Boston, MA: Beacon Press, 2006).

9. Boyle et al., "Effect of a Purpose in Life."

Chapter 24—It's Never Too Late

1. Dominique Mosbergen, "This Inspiriting Runner Took a Nasty Fall, But She Didn't Stay Down for Long," Huffington Post, accessed November 17, 2015, http://www.huffingtonpost.com/2014/05/27/runner-falls-wins-race-heather-dorniden_n_5395232.html.

INDEX

ABOUT DR. CAROL

CAROL PETERS-TANKSLEY, MD, DMin (known to many simply as Dr. Carol) is an ob-gyn, ordained Christian minister, and media personality. She has practiced medicine for over twenty years and is board certified in obstetrics-gynecology and reproductive endocrinology. With medical licenses in Texas, California, and Minnesota, she currently practices part time so as to devote more time to her writing, media production, and ministry. Throughout her career she has also regularly been involved in training medical students and ob-gyn resident physicians.

Dr. Carol received her medical degree from Loma Linda University and completed an ob-gyn residency at Loma Linda University Medical Center, Loma Linda, California. She completed a fellowship in reproductive endocrinology at Medical College of Georgia, Augusta, Georgia. Since 1992 she has practiced in many professional settings, including full-time university faculty, solo private practice, clinic and group practice, large county teaching hospital, and *locum tenens* (relief work).

While continuing to practice medicine, she completed an MDiv (master of divinity) and then a DMin (doctor of ministry) degree from Oral Roberts University, Tulsa, Oklahoma, focusing on Christian leadership. She subsequently founded Dr. Carol Ministries as a nonprofit Christian ministry dedicated to helping people discover the full and free life that Jesus came to give each one of us.

Dr. Carol and her husband, Al Tanksley, have been producing radio programs since 2009, and now the *Dr. Carol Show* is on television. She also enjoys speaking to church groups, women's groups, and doctors-in-training, among others. Check out www.drcarolministries. com for Dr. Carol's schedule, current program listings, blog articles, and more.

Dr. Carol and Al make their home in Austin, Texas, where she enjoys being Grandma Carol to four wonderful grandchildren.